Acclaim for
High Blood Pressure

"*High Blood Pressure: The Black Man and Woman's Guide to Living with Hypertension* is a coffee table reader to be shared with the family. Its text is easy to understand and offers a comprehensive overview of the importance of taking responsibility for your own health. ISHIB applauds Dr. Reed and Dr. Hudson for this important contribution. Read it – it can change your life."

– Kermit Payne, Executive Director
International Society for Hypertension in Blacks

"A very important book which will educate African Americans on the dangerous and deadly consequences of high blood pressure. Most importantly, African Americans will learn how to achieve the improved quantity and quality of life that result from good blood pressure control. The risk of heart attacks, heart failures, strokes, and kidney failure can be significantly reduced when blood pressure is controlled....A superb resource."

–Anne L. Taylor, M.D.
Associate Dean for Faculty Affairs, Professor of Medicine
University of Minnesota Medical School

"*High Blood Pressure* is a must read. It gives all the information you will need to take charge of your health. It...can save your life. A brilliant review of an illness that afflicts African Americans more frequently than all other races."

– Alphonso N. Goode, Executive Director,
Black Healthcare Initiative Coalition

High Blood Pressure

THE BLACK MAN AND WOMAN'S GUIDE TO LIVING WITH HYPERTENSION

JAMES W. REED, M.D., F.A.C.P., F.A.C.E. AND
HILTON M. HUDSON, II., M.D., F.A.C.S., F.C.C.P.

HILTON PUBLISHING COMPANY • ROSCOE, ILLINOIS

ISBN: 0-9716067-1-4

Hilton Publishing Company
PO Box 737, Roscoe, IL 61073
815-885-1070
www.hiltonpub.com

Notice: The information in this book is true and complete to the best of the authors' and publisher's knowledge. This book is intended only as an information reference and should not replace, countermand, or conflict with the advice given to readers by their physicians. The authors and publisher disclaim all liability in connection with the specific personal use of any and all information provided in this book.

Printed and bound in the United States of America.

Publisher's Cataloging-in-Publication
(Provided by Quality Books, Inc.)

Reed, James R., 1944–
     High blood pressure ; the Black man and woman's guide to living with
hypertension / by James R. Reed and Hilton M. Hudson II. — 1st ed.
     p. cm.
     Includes bibliographical references and index.
     ISBN 0–9716067–1–4

     1. Hypertension—Popular works. 2. African Americans—Diseases. 3. African Americans—Health and hygiene. I. Hudson, Hilton M. II. Title.

RC685.H8R44 2002   616.1'32'008996073
                                                   Qb102-2002284

CONTENTS

Dedication

This book is dedicated to Katherine, Mary, Robert, and David the brightest stars in my universe with hopes that they will live long, healthy, and prosperous lives. They have served as an inspiration for my efforts in educating the public about healthy life styles.

James W. Reed, M.D.

To my dad and mom, thank you for your love and unconditional support, and to Dr. P. David Myerowitz, a true embodiment of integrity, character, and honor.

Hilton M. Hudson, II, M.D.

Acknowledgements

Adrianne Appel's contributions can't be praised highly enough. Her intelligence and warmth are the voice of this book.

The authors and the publisher would also like to thank Pfizer Pharmaceuticals, Inc., for its gracious unrestricted grant in support of this project.

CONTRIBUTORS

Leo C. Egbujiobi, MD, FACC, FACP., is Chief of Cardiology at the Beloit Clinic, Beloit, WI.

John M. Flack, M.D., M.P.H., is a specialist in clinical hypertension, Professor and Associate Chairman for Academic Affairs, and Chief Quality Officer, Department of Internal Medicine, Wayne State University and the Detroit Medical Center, Detroit, MI. Dr. Flack is the current President of the International Society for Hypertension in Blacks (ISHIB).

C. Alicia Georges, EdD, RN, F.A.A.N, is affiliated with Herbert H. Lehman College, City University of New York, and is the current Secretary/Treasurer of ISHIB.

Hilton Hudson II, M.D., F.A.C.S., F.C.C.P. is a practicing heart surgeon and Vice Chairman of Cardiovascular Surgery, Rockford Health Systems, Rockford, IL.

James W. Reed, MD, F.A.C.P, F.A.C.E is Professor of Medicine and Associate Chair of Medicine for Research, Morehouse School of Medicine, Atlanta, GA. He is the co-founder of ISHIB.

Carmen Samuel-Hodge, Ph.D., RD is Co-Principal Investigator/Project Director of A New DAWN (Diabetes Awareness and Wellness Network), Center for Health Promotion and Disease Prevention, University of North Carolina, Chapel Hill.

Charles Washington, M.D. is a Clinical Instructor at the University of Illinois College of Medicine, Rockford, IL. He is Chairman, Department of Family Medicine, Rockford Memorial Hospital, Rockford, IL, where he also serves on the Credentials Committee. He is the president and founder of Whole Life World Ministries, a non-profit organization, is an ordained minister of the gospel of Jesus Christ, and is an active member of the St. Paul Church of God in Christ, serving as trustee board chairman.

INTRODUCTION

Health disparities, or inequalities, are a worldwide problem. Poor countries generally have weaker health services than rich ones. Thus in some countries people don't get the medicines they need, nor other forms of treatment and follow-through.

Similar disparities are a problem in the United States. Black people are more likely to fall ill, to get diagnosed later, to have less access to health care, and even to die from certain diseases than white people are.

Part of this problem is in the health care system itself. We don't mean to understate that. But what we want to tell you is what you can do to correct the problem. That means knowing what you need to know about your own health condition, and doing what you can to keep yourself well and to get early treatment when you need it.

High blood pressure is a perfect example of a health condition that each reader can work to improve. We want you to know

- how to avoid doing things that contribute to high blood pressure

- how to get yourself diagnosed by a doctor or other health care professional

- how to follow-up on treatment and on the practices you can adopt for yourself, like diet and exercise, and changing your life style

We want you to live a long and useful life and, by doing that, to change the statistics. High blood pressure, or hypertension, is a treatable disease. It's important for you to remember this fact. As it is now, too many of us, young and old, rich and poor, educated and not educated, are being struck down or disabled by heart attacks and strokes. Yet we can protect ourselves from a heart attack or stroke simply by taking the proper steps before a crisis occurs.

We wrote this book because we believe that in medicine, as in so much else, the truth can make you free. We wrote this book to dispel false beliefs about hypertension, such as the belief that there's nothing you can do to control it. In fact, there's much you can do, and we will tell you what that is.

Chapter by chapter, in simple, direct language, we tell you what a well-informed patient needs to know to stay healthy or get healthy if he or she already has high blood pressure. By learning what you need to know, you can better work with your doctor to become a partner in your own health. People who have a strong working relationship with their doctor are likely to get the best help and have the best chance for good health.

Taking care of yourself is something you do for yourself. It means taking pride in the life of the body you've been given, and treating that gift with the great respect it deserves. Taking care of yourself is also a way of telling your loved ones that you love them too. By living longer and setting an example of good health, you spread the word to others. You become a role model in your own right. People who take care of themselves are people ready to go on to realize their hopes and dreams. You can be one of them!

CHAPTER ONE

Understanding Your Blood Pressure

A diagnosis of high blood pressure is not something to fear. Changes in your lifestyle, in consultation with your physician, along with medication, can bring your blood pressure under control. To do this, the doctor may ask you to change your diet, quit smoking, lose weight, and check your own blood pressure regularly. You may need to take medication. All of this takes time, but longer life, with lower danger of serious vascular disease, is worth time and effort.

But to take these necessary steps you need first to understand what your blood pressure is, what happens when it gets too high, and how you can get the medical care you need in order to treat it.

WHAT IS BLOOD PRESSURE?

Blood pressure is the force of the blood as it moves through your arteries, or tubes that carry blood away from the heart. In a healthy person, blood pressure rises during exercise, or when one is scared or excited, but then returns to normal. But in someone who has a diagnosis of high blood pressure, it is high all the time.

There are two parts to a blood pressure reading, which is always expressed as "x over y." The top number, called *systolic pressure*, is the pressure in your artery that results when the heart contracts, or squeezes. The bottom number, called *diastolic pressure*, is the pressure in the artery when the heart is at rest, when it is relaxing. Doctors call an "optimal" (best possible) blood pressure 120/80 (that is, the systolic pressure is 120, and the diastolic is 80) . Normal blood pressure is 130/85 and "high normal" is 130-39/85-89. High blood pressure is a reading of 140/90 or higher – that is, the systolic pressure is 140 or above, the diastolic 90 or above.

In ninety-five percent of all people with high blood pressure there is no known cause. This is called *essential hypertension*. Essential hypertension can be made worse by stress, smoking, a diet high in salt, and too much weight. In a few cases, high blood pressure is the result of kidney disease, tumors, lead poisoning, or certain chemicals and drugs such as cocaine and crack and certain things we eat, such as licorice. This is called *secondary hypertension.*

SYMPTOMS

High blood pressure can cause headaches, dizziness, weakness, temporary blindness, chest pains, and nose bleeds. Left untreated, it can lead to stroke, heart attacks, kidney disease, blindness, leg ulcers, and loss of limbs. Or you may have absolutely no symptoms at all. That is why high blood pressure is sometimes called a "silent killer."

But a diagnosis of high blood pressure is hardly a death sentence. Rather, it is the opposite. Once you know you have high blood pressure, you can receive treatment and get your blood pressure under control.

> *High blood pressure can be treated.*

So, we urge you to consider the diagnosis a clear sign that you need to make changes in the way you have been living your life, and to seek medical treatment. If you haven't visited a doctor regularly, now is the time to start. Don't leave your life in the hands of fate but take it into your own hands.

THE DOCTOR'S VISIT

When you go to the doctor's office to have your blood pressure checked, be willing to ask questions. You need to know:

- what your blood pressure is

- how low it should be and how to bring it back into the safe range if it's high

- roughly how long it should take you to reach your goal

- the names of the drugs, or medications, you will be taking

- any diet or exercise suggestions

In most cases, your doctor will tell you these things. But you'll ensure the best treatment for yourself if you ask questions and write down the answers. (Bring a notebook with each of the above questions on blood pressure, diet, etc., written in advance on a single page, with room to write down the doctor's answers.) Doing this not only guarantees that he tells you everything you need to know, but also that he understands that you are the kind of patient who wants to take your health in your own hands, by asking questions and following instructions.

This same notebook in which you've recorded these questions and answers can become your blood pressure journal. Here you'll write down the several readings you take each day—say, one when you get up, one at lunch time, another in the evening before you go to bed. You will, in short, record your progress on the road back to good health.

Be sure to have your doctor or health care provider tell you how much and what kind of exercise you need, how much weight you should lose, and what types of foods to avoid. The doctor should also tell you what, if any, problems (which are called side effects) you might have from your medication. For most people, side effects are mild or unnoticeable.

You can achieve your goal with will power and the help of good medical care.

If you don't reach your blood pressure goal within the time discussed, talk with your doctor about what further changes you need to make in diet, exercise, or medication. *With attention, will power, and the help of good medical care, you can achieve your goal.*

It should be easy to motivate yourself. Just keep in mind that untreated blood pressure is a ticking bomb. Besides, you'll reap many benefits from bringing your blood pressure under control. Not only will you have a better quality of life, but you will feel better and have more energy. Remember, you owe this to yourself and to the family that loves you and needs you.

Involve your family members in the changes you are making. High blood pressure often runs in fami-

Involve your family members in the changes you are making.

lies, so by teaching your children to eat well and exercise more you will be showing them the way to a healthier life. At times they can be the main force in helping you to stick with an exercise program. Better still, get them into the exercise program with you. Let them help to prepare the healthy meals that you need for weight control. Show them you care about them by living a healthier lifestyle and helping them do so as well. If Mavis could change her life, you can certainly change yours.

MAVIS'S STORY

Mavis Parker is a fifty-five year-old office manager for a large insurance company. She is married and has two children—a son thirty years old, and a daughter twenty-five. Mavis was diagnosed with high blood pressure during her annual check up. "But Doc, I feel fine," she said. She couldn't believe it. But she remembered that her own father had died of a heart attack, caused by high blood pressure. That helped her take in the news.

Mavis' doctor, Dr. Lloyd, prescribed medication and told her to gradually lose ten pounds and cut back on salt. Well, Mavis was faithful about taking her pills, but she hardly knew what Dr. Lloyd meant when he said the word "exercise."

Exercising was not part of her life and never had been. When she grew up in New Haven, girls didn't play sports and were discouraged from being "too active." So, while Mavis found it pretty easy to cut down on fat (at least a little), Dr. Lloyd's suggestion about exercise went right to the back of her mind. Deep in her heart she felt that the new diet and pills would treat her high blood pressure and everything would be okay.

At her six-month checkup, she hadn't lost a pound and her blood pressure, though a little better, was still far from her goal. "I don't get it, Doc. I'm taking my pills every day." Dr. Lloyd shook his head. "Well that's fine, Mavis," he said. "The pills are important and they can do you a lot of good. But for them to do their work, you have to do yours. What about your exercising and diet?" Mavis had to admit that that part of the plan was not going so well. "You know, Dr. Lloyd," she said, "I've been using more canola oil in my cooking. You said that was safer. But I have to admit that it's hard for me to give up those fatty meats. And, well, about exercise, I just never was much for that."

Dr. Lloyd explained that if she didn't begin to exercise and eat less fat and salt, he would have to prescribe a higher dosage of medication to bring her blood pressure down, and that could mean she'd have side effects to deal with.

Mavis thought about her father's death again. How terrible the loss was to her and her mother, and what a tough time her mother had raising her alone. Mavis could hear her father telling her how important it was to make these changes. For herself. For her family. "This will be the start of something new," she told herself on the way home.

Mavis learned that two women she liked in her apartment went for walks each morning. She started going out with them, and before she knew it, her pressure was under control. Her new friends also told her how they'd been able to cut down on fat in their diet, and cut down on salt too, and how much better they felt now. Soon, with their help, Mavis was cutting down too. She got plenty of help. Everybody was telling her how great she looked, and she felt better than she had in years.

At first, her husband complained about the new diet. But she used spices instead of salt to liven things up and pretty soon they were enjoying the new food. Before she knew it, her husband was walking with her before breakfast. At first, their son and daughter were amused by all these changes. But after a while, they started to follow Mavis's example. As young as they were, with exercise, better diet, and shedding a few pounds, even they began to feel better than they had in years.

Remember, the best medical treatment really starts with you. When you start to make changes, the rewards will be yours for the taking.

> *Remember, the best medical treatment really starts with you.*

What we can learn from Mavis's story

- *You can feel fine but still have high blood pressure*

- *You can take control of your life*

- *Exercise and diet can help lower your blood pressure*

- *Feel proud of your success*

WHAT IS HIGH BLOOD PRESSURE?

High blood pressure is when your blood pressure is above normal. As you know, normal blood pressure is below 130/85. Your doctor will take three readings to determine if your blood pressure is safely within a desired range. If you have another condition such as diabetes, your doctor may want your blood pressure to be even lower than that, perhaps at the "optimal" level of 120/80.

The diagnosis of high blood pressure is based on your health history and two or more blood pressure readings on separate visits to your doctor. The diagnosis of high blood pressure is never made on only one reading.

If your blood pressure is not in the safe zone, your doctor will probably talk to you about bringing your blood pressure back down to a safe range. His role is to prescribe the medication, or drugs, you need, and to monitor the effect of the medication and diet and exercise on your blood pressure. Your role is to take care of yourself by watching what you eat according to a plan you've worked out with the doctor, getting as much exercise as your condition allows and the doctor recommends, keeping an eye on your stress, and with the help of counseling or in a support group, learning how to manage it better.

> *High blood pressure is based on your health history and two or more blood pressure readings.*

The following chart from the National Heart, Lung, and Blood Institute of the National Institutes of Health explains blood pressure levels:

CATEGORIES FOR BLOOD PRESSURE LEVELS IN ADULTS (AGES 18 YEARS AND OLDER)

Category	Systolic (mmHg)	Diastolic (mmHg)
Optimal	< 120	< 80
Normal	< 130	< 85
High Normal	130–139	85–89
High Blood Pressure		
Stage 1	140–159	90–99
Stage 2	160–179	100–109
Stage 3	≥ 180	≥ 110

(These categories are from the National High Blood Pressure Education Program of the Joint Commission for the Detection, Evaluation, Prevention and Treatment of High Blood Pressure.)

HOW TO TAKE YOUR OWN BLOOD PRESSURE

You may be asked to take your own blood pressure between visits to your doctor. To begin, you may need to purchase a stethoscope, the device the doctor uses to listen to your heart, and a sphygmomanometer, the cuff and bulb used to take your blood pressure.

There are a number of blood pressure kits available in pharmacies that carry medical equipment. They cost about $35. Ask the nurse if there's one kind that might be the best choice for you. If you are not comfortable taking your own pressure, you can ask a family member or friend to do it for you.

Another option is to buy an electronic device that takes pressure automatically. These are more expensive but they are simple and accurate.

To take your blood pressure:

1. Sit down and relax for five minutes.

2. Wrap the cuff around your upper arm, leaving about one inch between the bottom of the cuff and the bend in your elbow. Be sure that no clothing is caught under the cuff.

3. Hold the rubber bulb so that the screw lies between your thumb and forefinger. Inflate the cuff by squeezing the rubber bulb until you can no longer feel your pulse beat in your wrist. Write down the number you see on the gauge.

4. Turn the screw to the left, releasing the pressure, until the gauge reads zero.

5. Add 30 to the first number you wrote down and pump up the cuff until the gauge reads this number.

6. Place the stethoscope directly over the main artery of your arm, at the elbow bend.

7. Slowly release the air in the cuff and, using the stethoscope, listen for the first tapping sound. When

HOW BLOOD PRESSURE IS MEASURED

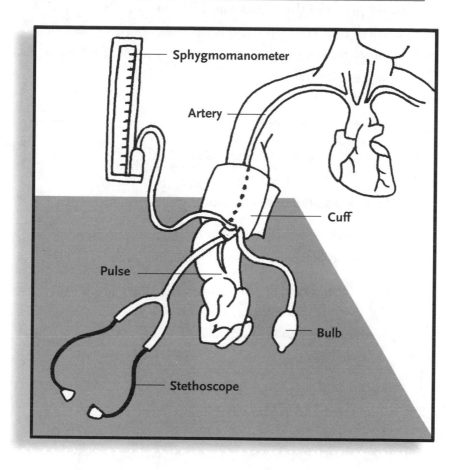

you hear it, note the number on the gauge and write that number down. This is your systolic pressure, the top number of the reading.

8. Keep listening until the tapping stops. Note this number. This is your diastolic pressure, the bottom number.

Remember to take your pressure three times. If you take your blood pressure three times and it is higher than your doctor recorded, or if your pressure is not getting lower over time, make an appointment with your doctor so you can find out why you are not getting better.

IN A NUTSHELL

- High blood pressure is a reading of 140/90 or higher.

- Blood pressure is controllable through medication and changes in lifestyle.

- High blood pressure often comes without symptoms, so it's very important that you see your doctor to have your book pressure checked.

- Before you leave your doctor's office you should know:
  – what your blood pressure is
  – if it's high, how low it should be
  – about how long it should take you to reach your goal
  – the names of the medications you will be taking
  – what kind of diet and exercise you should start

- Once you've been diagnosed with hypertension, you need to watch and check your own blood pressure.

- Tell your doctor about any big changes in your blood pressure readings.

CHAPTER TWO

High Blood Pressure Risks

John Johnson thanked the Lord that he had finally lost his stubbornness last year and went to see the doctor for a complete medical exam. He had health insurance from his former job at the steel plant. He was sixty-seven and retired, with a decent pension. John felt pretty good so hadn't seen any reason for going to the doctor. It was Bettina, his wife of forty-seven years, who finally made him go. "Look, John. I just want that doctor to put his stamp on you. Let *him* decide how healthy you are."

Once in Dr. Stilson's office, John told the doctor that he did have a lot of headaches, couldn't remember any time he hadn't had them, and figured it was from drinking too much coffee. "Well, maybe that's it, John, but I'd like to look into it a little further."

When Dr. Stilson asked John about his family history, he got an earful. "I grew up in Alabama, in a tin and wood shanty. My family all worked as crop sharers on a cotton farm, until my daddy died of a heart attack at forty-nine."

The doctor then began the exam by noting John's height

and weight, 5 feet 10 inches, and 250 pounds—more than a little overweight. Then Dr. Stilson reached for his blood pressure cuff and wrapped it around John's upper arm. He squeezed on the bulb and let the mercury fall. The doctor got a reading, but to be sure, several minutes later, he checked it a second time. John's blood pressure was 180/110, dangerously high.

"Mr. J," he declared in his booming voice, "You are an atomic bomb that could explode at any second!" John shrugged. He didn't think much of the reading, he mostly felt fine, and he told the doctor so, too. Dr. Stilson took John's words in stride. He had been through this many times with other older men. They felt all right and didn't want to believe that they could be weeks or even days away from a stroke or heart attack.

"You see, John, you are a lucky man. Your body is giving you a signal that you aren't in good health. That's what these numbers mean. The Lord is giving you a chance to listen and act." John said nothing but he sure was listening now. These were the best years of life for him and Bettina. He had no wish to lose them, and he sat quietly, though a little nervously, through the rest of the exam.

Continuing his exam, Dr. Stilson pressed with his thumb on John's lower legs. Where his thumb pressed, a dent was left, so he knew that John had mild swelling there. Dr. Stilson knew this was because of fluid that was building up in John's lower legs.

The doctor took a bright light and shined it into the center of John's eyes so he could look inside of his eyes and examine the blood vessels there. He saw changes that showed damage the high blood pressure had caused. Then Dr. Stilson put the end of his stethoscope on the arteries on the sides of John's neck and was able to hear the blood rushing through his arteries—not a good sign. In normal arteries he would not be able hear the blood flowing, so he suspected that these arteries also were damaged.

The doctor then moved the stethoscope to the left side of John's chest, so he could listen to his heart. There was a sound called a heart murmur, which meant that John might have damaged heart valves that were not opening and closing as they should.

Dr. Stilson finished his exam and John got dressed. Then they had a talk in the doctor's office. The doctor told John that he probably had high blood pressure for a number of years and that, as a result, it looked like his blood vessels and possibly his heart, too, were damaged. He was headed straight for a stroke, a heart attack or both. John had to get his blood pressure under control. Right now!

Dr. Stilson asked John about his diet. John still liked eating good down-home food: grits with bacon for breakfast, fried chicken and biscuits, a hamburger or a pork sandwich for lunch, and boiled salt pork or smoked ham hocks with vegetables for supper. Bettina made hot biscuits the way his mother did, served with butter and molasses. Every Saturday she made hot water corn bread, fried in hot grease. On Sundays in the summer, Bettina made John's favorite dessert, peach cobbler with a crust made from lard with the peaches floating in a heavy sugar syrup loaded with melted butter. John described Bettina's cooking with obvious glee.

Dr. Stilson sympathized. He once ate similar food himself, and he knew how good it was. But now, he told John, "You're going to have to do the same thing I did. You're going to have to cut out salt, grease, fried foods, and limit your butter."

"You also need to lose some weight and quit smoking," he told John. And he wanted John to go to the hospital where his heart and kidneys could be tested. "I never knew a man's life could change so much in one hour," John told the doctor as the two shook hands. John didn't know it then, but Dr. Stilson had saved his life.

What we can learn from John's story

- *Your doctor should give you a full and complete examination*

- *The examination can tell your doctor many things about your condition*

- *Your family, like John's, depends on, and needs you. So get your blood pressure under control for your sake—and for theirs.*

ESSENTIAL HYPERTENSION

Most cases of high blood pressure are called "essential hypertension," meaning there is no known exact cause. But we do know certain factors play a big role in making high blood pressure worse. When people eat diets high in salt, when they drink too much alcohol, when they don't get the exercise they need, their blood pressure may go up.

So your job is clear: Do what you can to eliminate the risk factors for vascular disease. You can

- go on a healthy diet and lose weight

- cut down on alcohol or, if you have alcohol problems, give it up altogether

- exercise regularly

- quit smoking

Eliminate risk factors and reduce your chance of hypertension.

As for salt, cut back for a while and see what happens to your blood pressure. If it goes down, you know that you are salt sensitive and should avoid it as much as possible. Removing risk factors reduces your chance of hypertension.

John could have been a poster boy for the risk factors for high blood pressure. He:

- ate a lot of salt and fat

- was overweight

- had lived a stressful life

- had a history of high blood pressure in his family (his father also had high blood pressure)

- smoked

It's also true that his being an African American was a risk factor because African Americans are especially at risk from this disease.

We will tell you more about these stress factors and how you can cope with them later in the book. We will also offer specific ways to change your diet and lifestyle and to get some relief from stress.

HYPERTENSION WITH KNOWN CAUSES

A small number of high blood pressure cases do have known causes. They are brought on as a result of another disease like cancer or kidney disease. This type of hypertension is called "secondary hypertension." In this book, we focus on the 95 percent of hypertension cases that have no known cause but get better when people eat a low-salt diet, get more exercise, and take any blood pressure medication their doctor may prescribe.

HYPERTENSION AND AFRICAN AMERICANS

High blood pressure is much more common and more severe among Black Americans. We don't know the exact reasons why this is so, but there are many ideas: stress, diet, social status, race and racial bias may all play key roles. As we say, these are only ideas, or theories, but some scientific evidence on these subjects is being gathered. For example, we know that Blacks in rural areas of Africa have lower blood pressures, which may rise when they move to urban areas. This suggests that stress or diet, not family history, is at the root of those cases.

Another factor that must be taken into account is that many Black Americans with less money and education don't have the chance to get regular health care. One of the great benefits of yearly physical exams is being able to catch diseases early, and this is especially true for high blood pressure. If caught early, blood pressure can be lowered and damage to organs prevented.

WHAT YOU NEED TO KNOW ABOUT SALT, SODIUM, AND FAT

Many studies have shown a link between high salt in the diet and high blood pressure. This is because salt contains sodium and sodium is processed by the kidneys. The kidneys help control blood pressure by holding more or less fluid in the body. When fluid builds up, blood pressure is higher.

The best information we have now tells us that reducing or limiting salt lowers blood pressure in only about one in three people in the general population. We think you should discover for yourself if you are salt sensitive. Limit your salt intake for a couple of weeks and see if your blood pressure falls. It's as simple as that. If it does, you know that you have a very strong reason to reduce the amount of salt you eat. Or talk to your doctor about other ways to discover if you are salt-sensitive.

For you and your family, reducing salt will mean eating less processed and fast food. Such foods rely heavily on salt for their "good flavor." You'll learn to use other spices instead of salt and serve foods with somewhat different flavors that will please your family in new ways, so you and they won't miss salt.

The recommended limit of sodium for the average American is 3,000 milligrams (mgs) per day, though some experts think that the recommended limit is too high, even for the average American who is healthy. These experts, doctors and dieticians, argue that people who eat this amount of salt each day are likely to get high blood pressure as well as other diseases like heart disease. In fact, the National Academy of Sciences has suggested a limit of 500 mgs of sodium per day as an amount that is safe for most people.

If you catch high blood pressure early you can lower it and prevent damage to organs.

People from other areas, such as those in rural parts of Africa, who eat low amounts of sodium have almost no high blood pressure.

But in America we eat a lot of salt. It is thought that many Americans eat between 2,300 mgs and 6,900 mgs of sodium each day. Keep in mind that one teaspoon of table salt contains 2,132 mgs of sodium! An order of Burger King fries has 1,110 mgs. of salt, or about one-third your 3,000 mgs recommended daily intake.

So, while the official recommended limit is 3,000 mgs per person, your own doctor or dietician may say that this is too high. If you have high blood pressure, your doctor will surely ask you to begin cutting back on the amount of sodium you take in.

Remember, sodium is found naturally in many fruits and vegetables in very low amounts, but in processed foods sodium runs high. Sodium is everywhere: fast foods, frozen foods, snacks, canned foods, store-bought desserts, cookies, and crackers. Your favorite tomato sauce, your favorite soup, even a can of "plain" white beans can have loads of salt. Thankfully, you can buy many of these foods in "low-sodium" varieties. So many people today are cutting back on salt, food companies have had to make these low sodium foods available. Remember, the label on the can or package tells you how much salt (sodium) is in the product. *Read the label.*

Eating just one fast food meal of a hamburger and French fries will give you much more salt than you should have—and that doesn't include the fat that's in many fast foods, which we'll talk about later. If, after a fast food lunch, you add a dinner with frozen or canned vegetables and, maybe, store-bought refrigerator cake, you and your family will be far above the recommended salt limit. Then, if you're like most Americans and sprinkle salt on your food, your daily intake of sodium will be even higher.

Remember, the label tells you how much salt is in the product.

Traditional soul food and downhome cooking are often made with lots of saturated fat and salt. They're partly what make greens taste so good! But these ingredients are bad for us. So what's the answer? One is to take your favorite recipes, replace the butter and lard with vegetable oil and just don't add salt. Ignore the instructions to add it. The food will taste different, but the superb natural flavors of the vegetables and meat will shine through. Delicious!

The real way to bring down the amount of salt you eat is to become a salt detective. You will have to avoid eating most processed foods, and to check the labels on the foods you do eat. You'll also have to stop adding salt at the dinner table. All that may sound really hard but it can be done—you'll be surprised at how many people are already doing it.

According to Samuel J. Mann, M.D. (*Healing Hyperten-*

sion, A Revolutionary New Approach. NY: Wiley, 1999. p. 191), potassium may also help lower your blood pressure. If you're eating enough fresh fruits and vegetables as part of your daily diet, you probably are getting all the potassium you need.

Remember too that fresh fruits and vegetables are a key part of your diet! Several studies suggest that many Blacks with high blood pressure have lower levels of calcium intake than whites do. You can get your calcium from greens, dairy products and also from certain fish such as sardines. If you're not getting potassium or calcium in your diet as you should, talk to your doctor about supplements.

Of course, the best plan is to involve your family in your eating plans. Why not start your children on the road to good health by showing them, through example, how to eat well? When you tell them that eating healthier will help keep them well, they will want to support you and know more. (See chapter 6 for more on this subject.)

EXERCISE AND WEIGHT

Studies show that many people with high blood pressure also weigh too much. Being overweight, even by a small amount, can mean higher blood pressure. And the opposite is true too: if you can lose a few pounds, you may lower your blood pressure and add years to your life. Eating fewer calories is one way to lose weight. Another is to burn more through exercise. The combination of fewer calories and more exercise is best.

Apart from weight loss, exercise itself can lower blood pressure and be a healthy outlet for stress. Exercise will help prevent heart disease and give you more energy. You may be able to reduce the amount of blood pressure medication you are taking by exercising regularly.

In the United States, a higher percentage of Blacks than whites are overweight. This is a national health problem, and pushes up the death rate among Blacks for many diseases. Some studies show Black women to be 40 percent more likely to be overweight than white women. Don't be among the statistics! Take up exercise—your life may depend on it. (See Chapter 6 for more about exercise.)

Regular exercise is as important to people who are salt-sensitive as to those who aren't. It helps lower your blood pressure. If you are salt-sensitive, you're best off doing light exercise like walking, as your doctor recommends. You also will want to cut back on your alcohol use and, if you are alcoholic, get sober. It will be worth it because you may live longer.

SMOKING

Your doctor will no doubt tell you that if you smoke, you must quit. The same goes for chewing tobacco. There are no good results of smoking, only harmful ones. It is just plain bad for your body and the quickest way to shorten your life. Though cigarette smoking is not a direct cause of high blood pressure, it is a risk factor for

- heart disease

- strokes

- clogged arteries (peripheral vascular disease)

- mouth, tongue, stomach, and lung cancer

Nicotine causes blood vessels to shrink—to become narrower—to constrict. Constriction of the capillaries (tiny blood vessels) may increase the heart's workload and strain the blood vessels. Also, some chemicals in cigarette smoke may affect the way that blood clots, making it more likely for a heart attack to occur. Chewing tobacco does have a direct effect on blood pressure. A substance in the tobacco directs the kidneys to hold onto sodium, causing the blood pressure to rise.

Since high blood pressure and heart attacks go hand-in-hand, you are taking a very big risk with your life by continuing to smoke, and that's before the risk of lung cancer! Smoking puts you at risk of heart disease. Your doctor may prescribe medications to help you quit smoking or chewing. There are "stop smoking" groups in almost every community in the United States that you can find through your local lung association. Once you quit, you will find plenty of support. Many restaurants have "no smoking" sections and some communities have made it the law that restaurants do so or be smoke free.

ALCOHOL

A little alcohol is fine but too much is bad for blood pressure and the body, mind, and spirit overall. How much is too much? Check with your doctor, but usually no more than one to two drinks per day is recommended.

Some studies show that a glass of wine can help prevent heart disease but be cautious here. Definitely do not drink if you have a history of alcohol abuse or liver disease. Even without such a history, it's best to talk with your doctor about how much alcohol is safe for you.

HOW MUCH GREATER IS THE RISK FOR SMOKERS OF DYING FROM A MAJOR DISEASE?

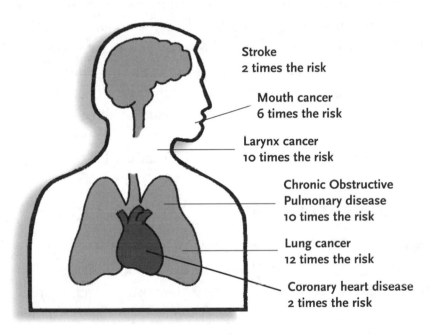

Stroke
2 times the risk

Mouth cancer
6 times the risk

Larynx cancer
10 times the risk

Chronic Obstructive Pulmonary disease
10 times the risk

Lung cancer
12 times the risk

Coronary heart disease
2 times the risk

Reprinted with permission from *The Black Man's Guide to Good Health,* by James W. Reed, M.D., F.A.C.P., Neil B. Shulman, M.D., and Charlene Shucker

FAMILY HISTORY

If your mother, father, grandparents, uncles, or aunts had high blood pressure, it is likely that this disease runs in your family. Your brothers and sisters should have their blood pressure checked regularly. So should you.

Will your children develop high blood pressure? Nobody knows for sure. But since you have high blood pressure, they are at risk and might get it too. The best way to make sure that they live healthy lives is to learn from you how to eat well, exercise, and visit the doctor regularly for blood pressure checkups. Make regular, healthy meals a family must in your household. If your family begins to eat healthy, low-fat, low-cholesterol, low-sodium diets, and exercises, you will be giving them a great gift—a longer and healthier life.

DIABETES AND BLOOD PRESSURE

Diabetes is common in the Black community and it often occurs together with high blood pressure. Both diseases affect the cardiovascular system, so when they occur together, they can be very dangerous. The Black community bears a much greater share of both diseases, so it is an important community health issue.

There are two types of diabetes, type I and type 2. Type I tends to develop from early childhood to young adulthood. But it can occur at any age. People with this type of diabetes tend not to be overweight, although there are exceptions. The cause of type I diabetes is not known. There really is no cure. Usually, a person with type I diabetes must take insulin each day in order to be able to process glucose, the simple sugar our bodies use for energy, and to sustain life.

Type 2 diabetes tends to develop among people who are overweight. It can sometimes be completely controlled through diet and exercise. In fact, the symptoms of type 2 diabetes can disappear, in some people, once they get down to a proper weight. Type 2 diabetes used to occur mainly among older, overweight Americans who did not exercise. Sadly, now even teens and preteens with poor eating and lifestyle habits are developing type 2 diabetes. Type 2 diabetes is two times as common among African Americans as in whites.

Diabetes and hypertension each carries huge risks, and even more so when they occur together. The risks from uncontrolled hypertension are the cardiovascular diseases we all fear:

- heart failure

- heart attacks

- strokes

- kidney failure

Many studies show that controlling high blood pressure reduces the risk of getting these complications by 35 percent to 65 percent.

The risks from uncontrolled diabetes are similar:

- heart attack

- stroke

- kidney failure

- loss of lower limbs, feet, or toes

- blindness

If the diabetes is controlled, these risks, too, can be reduced 35 percent to 75 percent.

As guardians of our own health, what must we do? Anyone who has not been checked for diabetes, must be checked. If diabetes runs in your family, be sure to tell this to your doctor. If you are overweight, even as a teenager, you should be checked each year for diabetes. If you are not overweight, you should be checked for it each year after you turn thirty.

If caught early, the most harmful results of diabetes can be prevented. Checking for diabetes usually involves a simple blood test.

If you have been diagnosed with diabetes there's much you can do. Poor diet and a lack of exercise contribute to the development of diabetes, and also to hypertension. Poor diet and lack of exercise also make it harder to control both diabetes and hypertension. So talk to your doctor about a diet that can help keep you well. If you are overweight, he'll probably want you to lose weight with diet and exercise.

Exercise is simple. A brisk walk of thirty to forty-five minutes each day is a great way to control diabetes and hypertension. If you're out of practice, start slowly with a walk that's easy, one that doesn't leave you panting. If you keep up that easy walk for a while, you'll get stronger and be able to keep going longer. Soon you'll find yourself doing several miles and enjoying it. Just remember to talk to your doctor or health care provider before starting any exercise program.

If you drink alcohol speak with your doctor. He may want you to reduce or stop your drinking.

Too many of us are dying needlessly because we fail to take our health in our own hands. Only you can control these diseases and help reduce the African America death rate. And only you can change your own lifestyle.

IN A NUTSHELL

- If you eat a lot of fatty foods and salt, drink a lot of alcohol, smoke, don't get exercise, are overweight, have uncontrolled diabetes, or aren't dealing well with stress, you're at high risk for hypertension.

- Too many Black Americans don't get the medical attention they need and that is available to them.

- Annual check-ups for you and your family can save lives.

CHAPTER THREE

Stress

Think about these stress facts:

- People who have chronic stress are 4.5 times more likely to die of heart attack or stroke

- Many adult visits to doctors are for stress-related illnesses

- Job stress in the United States, costs approximately $200 billion annually because of missed work, work that's not done well, and the cost of insurance claims.

- In a 1995 poll, seven of ten people interviewed said that they felt stress in a typical workday, and 43 percent said that they suffered physical and emotional symptoms of burnout

In Chapter 7 we're going to tell you the basics of stress relief. But first, let's think about stress.

LEANNE'S STORY

When Leanne Prout was told she had high blood pressure a year ago she became a good patient. Leanne was careful to watch her diet, exercise, and take her medication. And her blood pressure went down because of it. She was pleased. She'd gotten her health back, hadn't she? And she'd done it by taking charge of her life and making changes. It gave her a strong sense of pride.

There was a lot of excitement in Leanne's life at this time. After her last review at the office, she was told she'd soon have the chance for a better job. She was pretty sure that she was about to be offered the job of computer supervisor. She knew she was up for the work, but it would mean new duties and testing herself in a way she'd never been tested before. Along with the increased pressure, however, the new job would bring better hours and more pay, and that would mean having more time to spend with her little girl, Tina, whom she was raising on her own, and more money to buy the two of them what they needed.

Leanne waited. The job had been open now for three months and she had not heard a word. The longer she waited, the more she knew how badly she wanted the new job. She would be the first Black supervisor the company ever had. In the meantime, she said she would help plan the company's new computer system. She was putting in hours of overtime each week. The extra work was extra strain, but she felt good about it: it would show off her skills for her bosses to see.

That's what she was thinking about as she steered her car into the medical complex for her regular check-up, "Lord, I need this job, where is it?" Her health at this point was the last thing on her mind.

But when Dr. Farnum had finished his check-up, she knew even before he spoke that the news wasn't good. Yes, her blood pressure had gone back up, he told her. Together Leanne and Dr. Farnum went down the list to try to see what had changed in Leanne's routine. They crossed food, drink, medications, and exercise off the list. She'd been *very* careful about those.

Then he asked the big question, "What about stress, Leanne, has anything in your life been hard lately?" It didn't take long for Leanne to answer that one, "What? Stress? I've got nothing but stress!" Dr. Farnum suspected that Leanne's pent-up stress over the job had made her blood pressure worse. "You've gotten those other risk factors under control," he said, "and I know you can do the same with this one."

Doctor Farnum went over a list of ways that Leanne could cope with stress. When he came to "spirituality," Leanne lit up. Since she left her parents' home she'd lost touch with her spiritual side, and this was a great time to get back in touch with what had once meant a lot to her. She and the doctor worked out a plan—an experiment, he called it. Leanne would take five minutes to herself each morning for silent prayer. "I've seen it work many times," Dr. Farnum said. "Prayer seems to help people see more clearly, and understand that some things just aren't in our control. Those are the things," he said, "that the power we pray to can take over for us. Once you stop thinking that you can make everything happen as you want it and when you want it, I think you'll find that we'll have your blood pressure back under control again," he told her. After three months, the results were clear: Leanne felt calmer and her blood pressure had come down.

What we can learn from Leanne's story

- *Even if you try hard your blood pressure may not come down right away or it may go back up after you think it's under control.*

- *Many factors effect blood pressure*

- *Stress is one of the key causes of high blood pressure and hypertension*

- *Work out a plan to manage stress with your doctor*

- *Prayer and spirituality can help manage stress*

BLACK AMERICANS AND STRESS

You don't have to be the boss of a Fortune 500 company, or an airline traffic controller, or a heart surgeon, to experience stress. A bright young woman caught in a dead-end job, a single working mother trying to go to school at the same time, a father who rushes each day from work to pick up his daughter at day care—we have all felt it.

No matter where you live, or how, there's enough stress to go around. Stress hits everyone. It comes with our desire to perform well, to be better, and to do better. It comes with marriage and child raising. It's in our family relations and in our day-to-day efforts to be nice to others.

Yet, while everyone feels some stress, Black Americans often experience extra large portions. Sometimes racism and bias have been woven right into the fabric of the workplace, the schools, and the places where you do business. Sometimes, when your boss gives you a hard time, you may not be sure whether his harsh words are directed against the way you do your work or your skin color.

When you walk into a well-lit bank at noon to make a deposit for the company you own and the woman standing in front of you holds her purse closely, is it because she's nervous and would do this when anyone came up behind her, or because you are Black? In these cases what makes for unending stress isn't the certainty that you are being met with bigotry. It's the uncertainty.

HOW STRESS CAUSES HIGH BLOOD PRESSURE TO RISE

Stress is very closely linked to hypertension. Some doctors believe that pent-up stress worsens high blood pressure. How does that work? From the point of view of history, stress protects us. It lets the body rise to its highest level in response to some sudden danger. So it is when an otherwise calm female black bear turns savage because of a real or imagined threat to her cubs. So it is when a fish in a stream suddenly swims away, scared by your shadow. And so it is with you when, in an emergency, you see totally clearly and are able to do amazing acts as your body seems to say, "Let me handle this. We don't have time to think about it."

As soon as your brain senses something as a danger or fright, it gives the signal for your body to release two chemicals, epinephrine and cortisol. These chemicals prepare your body and mind to fight, run, and think fast. Epinephrine and cortisol are released by a small gland that sits on the kidney, the adrenal gland. Epinephrine is a powerful stimulant that jump starts your central nervous system, which causes your heart to beat faster and your breathing to quicken. Under stress, both epinephrine and cortisol will increase the speed at which your body responds to outside threats—your metabolism—causing the heart rate to increase.

Under stress, memory and thinking are usually better. Your thinking is sharper, clearer, and more precise. You breathe more quickly. Your heart beats faster and, as it does, your blood pressure rises. Your liver produces extra glucose, which creates more energy, so your heart beats faster and your pressure stays high.

Your pressure increases as your blood vessels squeeze tighter. They do this to increase the blood flow to important muscles used for running and fighting. When the vessels squeeze, blood pressure increases.

The constant reaction to stress puts your emergency stress system into overdrive. When it stays there, chronic high blood pressure can result.

This stress reaction is strong medicine, meant to be given only in real emergencies. When you are in danger, this medicine helps you rise to levels of effort you didn't think you had in you.

Normally, blood pressure goes back down after a stressful event. But some people's bodies react quite strongly to the stresses they face during the day. So the pressure stays high instead of coming back down. Some people, and you may be one, deal with many events each day that are deeply stressful. The constant reaction to stress puts their emergency stress system into overdrive. When it stays there, chronic, or long-term, high blood pressure can result.

A body can't go on at this high level without some bad symptoms, either physical or emotional, and often both. Stress can lead to high blood pressure, and more. (In Chapter 7 you will learn ways to lower the stress in your life.)

LONG-TERM STRESS HARMS THE BODY AND MIND

The chemicals the body releases during times of stress can cause the amount of fat and cholesterol in the bloodstream to rise. If your arteries are already damaged from high blood pressure, this extra fat and cholesterol can get stuck in the arteries and form plaque. If this plaque builds up to a point where it blocks an artery, it can lead to coronary artery disease, heart attack, and stroke.

Stress can get you into a kind of vicious circle. For some, higher stress means smoking more, or drinking more, or eating more. All of these habits increase the fat and cholesterol in the blood. Smoking, drinking too much, or eating, are just some of the ways that people try to cope with stress, but they don't work. The only real way to beat stress is to learn coping devices that do work.

Left alone, stress can weaken the immune system, the body's defense against getting sick. A study done at Carnegie Mellon University found that people with high stress were twice as likely to get colds. Why? Researchers think that the

DECREASED BLOOD FLOW TO HEART
MAY CAUSE HEART MUSCLE DAMAGE

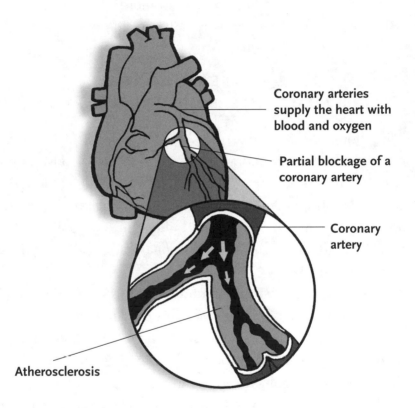

Coronary arteries
supply the heart with
blood and oxygen

Partial blockage of a
coronary artery

Coronary
artery

Atherosclerosis

CORONARY ARTERIES PROGRESSIVELY CLOSING (FROM LEFT TO RIGHT) AS A RESULT OF CORONARY ARTERY DISEASE

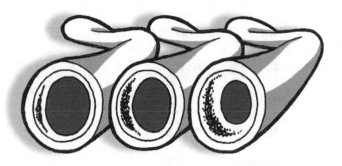

cortisol triggered by stress interferes with the ability of the white cells to fight off disease.

During stress, blood is sent away from the stomach and out to the arms, legs, and brain, where it is needed to help us run, fight, or think about how to save ourselves. Now it looks as if under chronic stress, this decreased blood flow to the stomach can lead to ulcers. The adrenal glands themselves suffer from the long-term effects of stress: The heavy discharges of cortisol can become poisonous, or toxic, when they are produced steadily.

There is new evidence that diabetes can result from chronic stress, as the body becomes less and less able to secrete insulin, a hormone that allows the cells to absorb glucose, the simple sugar the body uses for fuel.

People who are stressed often don't even realize it. Here are some signs:

THE SIGNS OF STRESS

- Weight gain or too much weight loss

- Diarrhea or constipation

- Sleeplessness

- Headaches

- Sexual problems

- Drugs, too much drinking or gambling

- Smoking

- Anxiety

- Anger

- Depression or feelings of worthlessness and lack of satisfaction

- Forgetfulness

- Reduced creativity

- Inability to concentrate

Healthy people find ways to turn stress, and even fear, into superb performance. They take these so-called "negative" feelings and use them like rocket fuel to make positive needed changes in their lives or relationships. They know how to read the signs. If you are angry all the time, for instance, this may be a sign that you are in a bad situation, perhaps a dead-end job or a relationship in which the other person takes more than he or she gives. Your anger tells you that something has to change.

> *Healthy people find ways to turn stress, and even fear, into superb performance.*

Even if you aren't used to keeping tabs on your own feelings, you can begin now. If you are angry, ask yourself why. Make a list of possible reasons and explore them. Once you have an idea of what the problem is, talk to a friend or loved one you trust, somebody who isn't part of the problem. Your goal is to come up with a plan that will let you either change the situation or, if it can't be changed, let you find a healthy way of relieving stress.

Stress can be managed. It can be dealt with. But some people feel crushed by the stress in their lives. Maybe that is how you feel. Maybe you have the same amount of stress as your neighbor Ned, but Ned somehow deals with it better than you do. Chances are that Ned has found effective ways to let go of his stress and make it work for him. Maybe it's time for you to learn those ways. As it is now, you worry all the time, find yourself snapping at the people you love, or start each day with dread, instead of joy. As if all that weren't bad enough in itself, feeling this way all the time has a direct effect on your blood pressure!

Human beings are not built to go through life in a state of constant anxiety, anger, or fear. We were made to be happy, relaxed, and thoughtful, with some bouts of worry and anger. If any of the warning signs of stress ring true with you, begin to take some time to deal with stress. You'll feel better and happier, and you'll be taking one big step toward lowering your blood pressure.

BEING BLACK AND FEELING ALONE

Black Americans often feel the stress of being totally alone when we are outside our home communities, that is, away from our neighborhoods, churches, families, or our best friends. You may feel isolated, or alone, at work, in the classroom, on the street, in shops, or in the boardroom. You may feel uncomfortable being the only African American on the train, the only African American at work, the only African American in the grocery store.

The reality of life can certainly be harsh, but some people do learn to deal with such feelings in a way that doesn't make bad matters worse. It's important for your health to learn to cope with being Black. People who almost always feel uncomfortable or on the outside when they aren't in the company of other Black folks, experience continual stress. They may also become terribly isolated because they avoid conditions that will put them at risk of feeling cut-off from their own. They withdraw from their lives, which can lead to depression and more isolation. It becomes a vicious circle. Feeling isolated is a form of stress. And when there is stress, there is high blood pressure.

Yes, dealing with racism and the daily wounds we experience because of it can be a big challenge. But you can accept the challenge by seeing it as just one more form of stress that you must learn to cope with. (For help on this, see Chapter 7.)

CHRONIC STRESS
AND MENTAL HEALTH

Chronic, or long-term stress affects the way we think—or don't think. Anger, tiredness, and worry weaken our mental functions. Thus, the way we often see African Americans on television as angry or uptight, has a grain of truth in it. It's not because we are born that way, but because chronic stress can often lead to such emotions.

CONCEIT IS A FAST
WAY TO BECOME ISOLATED

Another way to stress yourself out is to be very self-absorbed, or into yourself, otherwise known as conceit. Studies of heart patients at the University of California at San Francisco found that they were especially likely to use pronouns such as I, me, and mine. Too much of this takes you straight down the road to social isolation and perhaps high blood pressure. People who think too highly of themselves—egotistical people—are more likely than others to feel apart from others, and they're also quicker to show hostility and anger.

So maybe it pays to keep the ego in check. The good, the generous, and the happy tend to live longer than the nasty and self-absorbed.

STRESS AND GRIEF

A different type of stress results from grief, above all when a relationship ends, or a loved one or lifelong partner dies. The feelings of being left totally alone can be so stressful as to force blood pressure to rise or to cause an overall downturn in one's health. In general, married people are healthier than people who never married, are divorced, or widowed. Studies have shown that after a husband or wife dies, it is not uncommon for the one left behind to die soon after, even though that partner had been thought to be in good health. It's not just in fairy tales that people die of broken hearts. In real life, too, grief and loss—and isolation—can result in high blood pressure, heart disease, and a higher death rate.·

Naturally, the most effective cure for isolation is to get involved with family and friends and social groups. Here, what common sense tells us is the best guide. We weren't made to be alone.

DEPRESSION AND HIGH BLOOD PRESSURE

Depression is closely linked to stress and, like stress, can lead to high blood pressure. The reason is that a depressed person will experience unusually high levels of cortisol, the hormone related to stress, and this can cause blood pressure to rise. Depression can result when we are faced over and over again with stress and isolation to the point where we just can't cope anymore. When we can't cope, it causes us to have feelings of worthlessness, making it even harder for the person to deal with his or her life. The depressed person may turn to addictive drugs, alcohol, stimulants, or even food for the satisfaction he or she lacks elsewhere. Of course, those alternatives don't work, and sometimes end up adding addiction to the problems the person already faces.

In the African American community depression tends to be overlooked and under-reported, in part because it's often seen as a sign of weakness or as a sign that the victim has lost faith in God or in life itself. These reasons, sometimes combined with the awful impact of poverty and the lack of knowledge that can go with it, mean that in the African American community stress and depression too often go untreated. That's too bad, because with the help of counseling and, sometimes, medication, depression can now be treated effectively.

SOME SYMPTOMS OF DEPRESSION

- Irritability and long-term, chronic fatigue

- Sleeping too much or too little

- Heavy use of, and need for alcohol and drugs

- Inability to concentrate

- Feelings of worthlessness and guilt

- An inability to act, even when action is necessary

If you suffer from any of these symptoms or a combination of them, and can't seem to shake them, seek help. Your spiritual congregation may provide counseling. Or your doctor can refer you to a psychologist. Your doctor can also talk to you about the kinds of medications there are and, if appropriate, send you to a specialist who will prescribe the right medication for you.

Finally, there are things you can do for yourself. Exercise can be very effective against depression. You can start at any level. In the beginning, by keeping your goals modest—say, by walking twenty minutes each day—you can begin to feel like you've done something special. You'll be surprised. This feeling might just start spilling over into other parts of your life.

Too few African Americans have taken advantage of these effective ways to be happier, more productive, and healthier. You can break that trend.

A WORD ABOUT STRESS AND ADDICTION

We all know people, even family members, who react to stress by turning to alcohol, drugs, too much gambling or shopping, too many sexual partners, or other addictive behaviors. We know promising and productive people who mysteriously slip, crash, and end up as drug addicts, alcoholics, or prostitutes, while their brothers and sisters lead successful lives. The reason actually is not so mysterious. These people do not know how to handle the stress in their lives, past and present.

Try to recognize the stress in your life and why it is present.

Try to recognize if the stress in your life and why it is there. Do something about it. Read and understand more about it, pray, exercise, talk with family and friends, or meditate. Take a step forward to change your life and reduce the stress! The courage and confidence to take the next step will quickly follow but you must take the first step—you owe it to yourself and your family!

IN A NUTSHELL

- People who are always stressed out are more likely to develop hypertension and other illnesses.

- Being Black in America is stressful, but you can cope with this stress.

- Heavy smoking, heavy drug or alcohol use, sleepless-ness, anger, depression, and forgetfulness can all be the signs of long-term, chronic stress.

- Prayer, meditation, and other forms of spiritual prac-tice can reduce stress.

- Regular exercise can reduce stress.

- Staying in contact with other people or even with pets will help you manage stress—even the stress that comes from the end of a relationship or the death of a loved one.

CHAPTER FOUR

Complications

Francis Tate enjoyed his life. He was married to the love of his dreams, Claudia, and he was the best car salesman in Tampa. He had a house on the bay with a deck, and Tuesday nights, his night off, his mother, sisters, and uncle came over for ribs. It hadn't always been like this: he had worked hard to get out of what looked like an endless pit of bills—and alcoholism. "Lord, how lucky I am!" he often told himself. But now, he thought, his troubles, and his struggles, were safely behind him.

So, when his doctor told him he had high blood pressure, possibly due to the alcoholism, and gave him a new diet and an exercise plan, he hardly gave it a second thought. "No Tuesday ribs? And exercise time to work into my day? No way am I going to give up the ribs or waste my time in a gym!" he told himself as he left the office. He kept the diagnosis to himself.

Francis had been having dizzy spells, but he told himself that was from drinking too much bad coffee. The tingling feeling in his right leg, he told himself, was a pinched nerve.

It went on like that for nearly a year when one day, just before he left the house for work, Francis fell. He got back on his feet, but then he was hit with a raging headache. When Claudia came into the room to see what had happened, he couldn't talk and just stood there, holding his head. That was the last thing he remembered. When he came-to he was lying in a hospital bed. Francis had just had a stroke.

The right side of his face was numb and he couldn't move his mouth. The doctor told Claudia that with therapy Francis might get some movement back on that side of his face but the outcome of the therapy was not certain.

When the doctor had explained this, he asked Francis, as gently as he could, whether Francis had known before the stroke that he had high blood pressure. Francis sighed, "Yes, doctor, I knew but I didn't listen."

Uncontrolled blood pressure can lead to strokes, kidney failure, and blindness. So take your diagnosis seriously.

Had Francis listened to the doctor who first diagnosed high blood pressure, his stroke might never have happened. Uncontrolled blood pressure can lead to strokes, kidney failure, and blindness. So take your diagnosis seriously. Only by taking care to diet, exercise, and follow the treatment plan your doctor has recommended for you can you protect yourself from the very serious health threats that may follow from uncontrolled high blood pressure.

What we can learn from Francis's story

- *Don't be afraid of, or ashamed of, having high blood pressure.*

- *Do something about your hypertension. Don't let it get worse.*

- *Listen to your body. Tell the doctor about any symptoms you have. And follow your doctor's advice.*

- *High blood pressure may cause stroke.*

HOW HIGH BLOOD PRESSURE CAUSES DAMAGE

How does high blood pressure cause such a huge problem? By blocking blood vessels and, over time, damaging and destroying them. Remember, high blood pressure can destroy the inner lining of the blood vessel, causing the artery to be blocked, much as a water pipe can become plugged with debris.

When blood vessels fail to work, parts of our body fail to get the nutrition they need. Blocks can occur anywhere—in vessels that feed the brain, heart, kidneys, eyes, and legs. So any part of the body can be harmed by weak and damaged blood vessels.

STROKE

A stroke occurs when an artery (a type of blood vessel) to the brain becomes clogged with fatty deposits. That part of the brain begins to starve from the lack of blood, oxygen, and nutrients. If not treated quickly, that part of the brain may die, resulting in a stroke. A large stroke can kill. These are called occlusive strokes. Hemmoragic strokes hit hard too and are more directly related to hypertension.

Strokes are twice as common in Blacks as in whites, and the death rate from strokes among Blacks in the United States is the highest in the world!

The figures on stroke and African Americans are grim: Strokes are twice as common in Blacks as in whites, and the death rate from strokes among Blacks in the United States is the highest in the world!

Strokes are more common in people older than forty-five, but they can and do occur in people as young as thirty-three.

It is not known exactly how high blood pressure causes strokes. The belief is that when the walls of the arteries to the brain are damaged from high blood pressure, the lining of the arteries becomes scarred. Fats in the blood get stuck to the scars. Over time, the fats, cholesterol, and other substances, like platelets, build up. Over time, the artery becomes so clogged that blood can no longer flow through, and a stroke results.

Of course, weak arteries are just one part of the issue. Having excess fat and cholesterol in the blood is the other. This

HOW CHOLESTEROL FORMS
ON THE WALL OF AN ARTERY

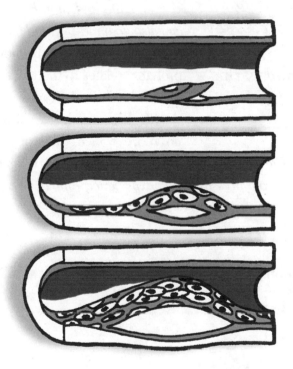

is why it is so very important that if you have high blood pressure, you limit the amount of fats and cholesterol you eat and be tested often for high cholesterol and fats in the blood.

weak arteries are just one part of the equation. Having excess fat and cholesterol in the blood is the other

Heavy drinking increases the amount of fats in your blood. This is yet another reason that people with high blood pressure shouldn't drink.

Smoking and high blood pressure can also go hand-in-hand with strokes. Why this is is not exactly known, but it probably relates to the fact that smoking tends to harm arteries.

Strokes may be small and cause no more notice than dizziness and numbness. Or they can be massive, causing coma or death. *If you have high blood pressure and experience any of the following symptoms, contact your doctor or emergency room immediately:*

- dizziness

- numbness

- loss of vision

- loss of balance

- temporary blindness

- loss of movement

- severe headache

- nausea and vomiting with a headache

- change in the way you speak

KIDNEY DISEASE

Kidney disease among Blacks is almost an epidemic. While 12 percent of the population of the United States is African American, nearly 30 percent of those with very serious kidney disease are Black. And, just as bad, Blacks with hypertension are more likely to develop kidney disease than whites with hypertension. Nobody knows the reason for this difference. It may be due to poor health care or the wrong medications, lack of knowledge about kidney disease, lack of knowledge about symptoms, poor access to medical care, or lack of follow-through with treatment. Whatever the exact reason for the difference, *it is essential that you ask your doctor to check how well your kidneys work.* This can be done through simple blood and urine tests.

Of course, the best way to prevent kidney disease is to eat a healthy diet and take the medication the doctor has prescribed for you to help lower your blood pressure!

HOW THE KIDNEYS FAIL

Kidneys help rid the body of wastes. Like the heart, kidneys need blood and oxygen to work. When the small arteries that carry blood to the kidneys thicken and narrow, and become damaged by high blood pressure, the arteries can get so clogged they no longer carry enough blood to the kidneys. The result is that the kidneys starve, shrink, and become damaged.

While there may be no symptoms other than having to go to the bathroom more, toxins build up in the blood and other organs and the kidneys begin to spill protein and sugar into the urine. That is, the kidney loses its function.

Often it is only when two-thirds of the kidney is damaged that a person begins to get headaches, weakness, nausea, and loss of appetite. Without a diagnosis and treatment, the kidneys can completely fail before you realize you are ill. Once they fail, the person must undergo dialysis, or weekly blood cleansing with an artificial kidney machine, in order to live. This is called *chronic kidney failure.* It is usually a gradual process but can often lead to other problems and death.

In *acute kidney failure,* the kidneys suddenly stop working. In this case, the kidneys are weak but the condition probably has not been diagnosed. When the person stresses the kidneys, which can happen by taking a simple drug like ibuprofen, the kidneys fail. Therapy can sometimes help the kidneys to work again.

Untreated high blood pressure can lead to kidney disease and you will never know it. Kidney failure is a bad problem that often involves the whole family and can bring about a very poor quality of life both for the ailing person and the family. Treat your high blood pressure and avoid developing kidney disease!

HEART DISEASE

Your heart is a muscle. Just like a muscle in your upper arm, the heart contracts (squeezes) and relaxes. The difference, of course, is that your heart contracts and relaxes many times a minute, which is how it pumps the blood throughout your body. In order to do its job, the heart requires oxygen and nutrients—vitamins, minerals, and simple sugars—that it gets from the blood.

High blood pressure is very hard on the heart. It causes the heart to grow larger than normal and can destroy the arteries around the heart. That is, high blood pressure can and often does lead to coronary artery disease, or hardening of the arteries.

High blood pressure and coronary artery disease go hand-in-hand. Many people with high blood pressure, and especially African Americans, also develop coronary artery disease and heart trouble. If you have high blood pressure, you are at much higher risk for heart disease than others. Prevent it from developing by eating well, exercising, and getting regular medical checkups. And, most importantly, control your blood pressure even when you feel well.

Many people with high blood pressure, and especially African Americans, also develop coronary artery disease and heart trouble.

How heart disease happens is similar to how a stroke happens. High blood pressure weakens and damages the arteries of the heart, making the arteries' walls flabby and causing scarring and narrowing . (This can happen to arteries anywhere in the body, even those leading into the heart.) Fats and cholesterol become stuck in the walls, forming a plaque, which makes it more difficult for blood and oxygen to flow to the heart. The arteries become clogged, like a plugged up pipe, or the plaque may suddenly rupture, plugging up the arteries (which is what happens most often). Without enough oxygen and nutrients, your heart may weaken, or parts can die. When the arteries that feed the heart are plugged up, the heart doesn't get enough blood.

The symptoms of heart disease are chest pain and pressure in the chest (called *angina*). Angina usually occurs in the center of the chest, but the symptoms can go out to the arms, throat, back and upper abdomen. It often feels like a heavy weight on the chest, like a bad case of indigestion.

Angina can be a warning sign that your heart is not doing well and it should be taken very seriously. Have a relative or friend call 911 right away and then call your doctor. Don't worry about being wrong and not having had an attack. Better to be proven wrong and be alive than wait!

Other symptoms of heart trouble include:

- shortness of breath

- fainting

- swelling of the legs

- nausea

If you have had uncontrolled blood pressure, make sure your doctor checks your heart as well as your levels of fats and cholesterol.

Over time, if treatment is not started, your heart can become so starved of oxygen and nutrients that it stops working. That is when a "heart attack" occurs. It is usually possible to recover from a heart attack if it is caught in time. But, as anyone who has had one will tell you, the road to recovery can be hard. If you have had uncontrolled blood pressure, make sure your doctor checks your heart as well as your levels of fats and cholesterol. It is your duty to know the signs of angina and heart attacks and to educate your family also. Your life depends on it!

CONGESTIVE HEART FAILURE

High blood pressure can also lead to congestive heart failure, a common reason for hospital admission. When you have high blood pressure, your heart pumps harder and more forcefully because it is more difficult to push blood through smaller, and often thicker, blood vessels. Over time, this can cause the heart to grow bigger and become less efficient at its job. To make up for this, it beats more and becomes very tired.

When your heart is tired, you feel tired. You feel tired all the time and find it difficult to breathe when walking or exercising. You may gain weight and look puffy in your face and legs.

Congestive heart failure is treated by lowering blood pressure and making the heart stronger, through medication, light exercise, and a low-salt, low-fat diet.

The major point here is that this can all happen without your knowing it. Therefore, always measure your blood pressure!

LEG ULCERS AND BLINDNESS

Just as high blood pressure narrows the arteries going to the brain and the heart, the arteries going to the eyes and lower legs are also narrowed. Remember, all the arteries in the body are affected by high blood pressure. As blood flow to the legs and eyes become less, leg ulcers and blindness can result. This is especially true if you have high blood pressure and diabetes. The more severe the blood pressure is and the longer it goes untreated, the more likely it is that leg ulcers and blindness will occur.

A LAST WORD

The lessons of this chapter are clear and important. You can develop serious complications if you don't know you have high blood pressure and don't get it treated. By seeing your doctor for regular check-ups, you can spot problems early and, with the help of good diet, exercise, and medication if necessary, you can correct them.

IN A NUTSHELL

- Uncontrolled hypertension can lead to blocked arteries and serious damage to many parts of the body, including the brain and the heart.

- Symptoms of heart disease include shortness of breath, fainting, swelling of the legs, nausea.

- Stroke can result from blocked arteries to the brain.

- Arteries get blocked by fat in the blood.

- If you're dizzy or have numb arms, legs, fingers or toes this may be a sign of stroke, See your doctor if these symptoms last for more than a few days.

In A Nutshell, *continued*

- Other symptoms of stroke include loss of vision, loss of balance, loss of movement, temporary blindness, severe headache, nausea, or changes in the way you speak. If you have any of these symptoms, see your doctor right away.

- Black Americans are more likely than White Americans to develop serious kidney disease, sometimes as the result of uncontrolled hypertension.

- Regular visits to your doctor that include tests of your kidneys can help keep you from suffering serious kidney disease.

- Congestive heart failure happens when your heart gets weakened by uncontrolled hypertension and is forced to work harder.

- By seeing your doctor regularly, you can spot these and other heart-related problems early, and, with the help of good diet, exercise, and medication if necessary, bring them under control.

CHAPTER FIVE

Drugs for Hypertension

Based on your health history and your blood pressure, your doctor may prescribe one or more medications to lower your blood pressure. It is very important that you tell your doctor about any other medical conditions you have so that the right drug is prescribed for you. Also be sure to tell the doctor about any other drugs you are taking, including non-prescription drugs like aspirin, diet or allergy pills, and any herbal remedies. While over-the-counter products are freely available and usually safe, they may be harmful when taken with certain prescription medications.

The key point is to always take your blood pressure medication, even if you are feeling great. If you want to stop taking your medication for any reason, first discuss it with your doctor. If you are having side effects from your blood pressure pills and this is the reason you want to stop taking them, tell your doctor. Many drugs are available to treat high blood pressure and there may be others you can take that will be easier for you. Remember, blood pressure medications are an excellent and effective way to treat and control high blood pressure. But

> *Tell your doctor about any other medical conditions you have so that the correct drug is prescribed for you. Also be sure to tell the doctor about any other drugs you are taking, including non-prescription medications like aspirin, diet pills or allergy pills, and any herbal remedies.*

never stop taking you medication without your doctor's approval.

Many blood pressure medications are available today. The ideal one for you will lower your blood pressure while keeping unwanted, and infrequent, side effects to a minimum. The doctor, nurse, or pharmacist should talk to you about these side effects when the drug is prescribed. Be truthful with the doctor or nurse. Unless they are treating you directly for other illnesses, they may not be aware of any problems you have unless you tell them yourself. Remember: most medications have few, if any, noticeable side effects. In general, the advantages of taking medications far outweigh these minor effects.

Another important note of caution is that you should never take anyone else's blood pressure drugs—neither your husband's nor your wife's nor a relative's. This is because each drug is chosen for each person based on his or her health profile. You risk having dangerous side effects by taking someone else's blood pressure pills. *If you have high blood pressure but have not been treated because you do not have health insurance, visit your local clinic. The staff there may be able to help you receive free or low-cost medication.*

When you get your drugs from the pharmacy, ask for an

information sheet about that drug. The sheet will tell you how to take the medication. If it is easier for you, ask the pharmacist to review it with you. This is part of her job.

To help you learn about some of the medications your doctor may prescribe, we will talk about common blood pressure medications and their possible side effects below. Once again, do not stop taking your medications without your doctor's okay, and always take your medications exactly as prescribed. If taken the correct way they are very effective.

If you respond well to your medication and you have made changes in your diet and lifestyle, the doctor may, over time, lower the prescribed dosage or take you off the drug altogether. This may be a goal for you. Discuss this goal with your doctor so you can come up with a plan for getting there.

SIDE EFFECTS AND ANTIHYPERTENSIVE DRUGS

Not only patients, but many physicians as well report symptoms like being tired and unable to stand exercise when they take drugs to lower high blood pressure. Such symptoms may be caused by the antihypertensive medication prescribed.

Drugs relieve far more side effects than they cause.

In our own clinical experience this is not the case. Hypertension itself causes these symptoms and the drugs relieve far more side effects than they cause. Clinical studies that have measured side effects in drug-treated patients support this view. Overall, people with hypertension feel better and report fewer side-effects as their blood pressure is slowly reduced with medication.

This does not mean that antihypertensive medication cannot make you feel bad. When your blood pressure has been high and begins to come down you may feel bad for a short time if the medication works very fast on you. Remember that even if you have some brief discomfort, the medication is doing its work.

Just keep the main point in mind: you will feel better, over the long-term after your body becomes used to the lower blood pressure. In most cases, then, the best advice when you feel bad after starting or increasing your blood pressure medication is to know that the bad feeling will pass and to keep taking your medication as prescribed.

A similar situation may happen when you take antihypertensive drugs but your blood pressure levels remain high. It is commonly supposed in this situation that reported symptoms are side effects of the drug. In most cases, though, the high blood pressure is more likely the cause. Again, changing or stopping medication(s) may not be the answer. Usually, the best way to handle this situation is to increase the antihypertensive treatment.

While your best course is usually to put up with the side effects until they pass, it is essential that you tell your doctor about any side effects you may have. Don't be shy! The doctor needs to know how you are feeling in order to know that the drug is working for you. If the drug is giving you any unwanted symptoms that linger, it may be possible to change the dose or switch you to a drug that will be easier on your body. The more you talk to your doctor, the more you will ensure that you are given the best drugs for treatment of your hypertension.

HOW MANY BLOOD
PRESSURE DRUGS TO TAKE

Many people with hypertension may need to take more than one drug to control their blood pressure. We are often asked, "Am I taking too many blood pressure medications?" The answer is not exactly straight-forward. The number of blood pressure drugs (along with other medications) can be a mental, or psychological, as well as a financial, barrier to achieving good blood pressure control. A good rule of thumb is that if your blood pressure is above your target level then usually, though not always, you will need to take more than one blood pressure pill. However, this isn't always the case.

Which drugs your physician prescribes will influence the number of antihypertensive drugs that you take. Some drugs work better together to lower blood pressure than others. It is, for example, a good idea to take a water pill (diuretic) when you are taking at least two other non-diuretic drugs but have not reached your goal blood pressure.

You and your physician(s) need to be patient when trying to find out if the medications you are taking have controlled your blood pressure. It takes at least four, and sometimes up to eight weeks after starting an antihypertensive drug for it to work best. Thus, you can not know if a drug or drugs are working well by changing the dose and/or medications prescribed every couple of weeks.

If you change your medications too often you will probably end up on too many of them and may find it hard to really achieve the blood pressure level you want. We have also found that rapid (every two weeks) increases in blood pressure med-

ication doses result in worse side effects compared to less fre-
quent (every six weeks) dose adjustments.

SHOULD RACE INFLUENCE THE SELECTION OF ANTIHYPERTENSIVE DRUG TREATMENT?

There is no reason to prescribe different antihypertensive
drugs to people of one racial or ethnic group than to another
group. What is crucial here is that your doctor prescribe high
blood pressure drugs for you that match your own needs. If you
have weak kidneys, for example, certain drugs may be safer for
you than others. Each drug interacts with the body in its own
way, and only your physician, who knows all your medical history, can choose the one that gives you the best chance to live
a long and active life.

REMEMBER TO TAKE YOUR PILLS

Remembering to take pills every day is not easy for everyone. If
you have a hard time with this, keep at the front of your mind that
the drugs are needed to bring your blood pressure under control
and to reduce your chance of having bigger health problems: a
heart attack, congestive heart failure, a stroke, kidney disease, or
death. That should be good motivation.

You may find it easier to remember when to take pills if you

- Take them at the same time each day. Write the time in
  a daily calendar. Or, set your watch alarm to go off at
  the time that you need to take your pills. Sometimes, it

works to take them before or after meals, as your doctor prescribes.

- Keep the pills in the same place (a kitchen cabinet, a night table by your bed, or in the bathroom, or, if they go with meals, at the place where you eat), so you see them every day and don't have to hunt around for them. This is extra important in case of an emergency. If you keep your pills in a particular place you can tell someone else, your family or a friend, where to find them. If you travel, it is useful to get a pill box with spaces for each day's dosage.

Try to memorize the names of the drugs you are taking. You may want to write them down and keep this paper with you, in your purse or wallet, so that in case of an emergency, health personnel will know that you have been taking blood pressure medications. Include in your list allergy pills, asthma inhalants, water pills, laxatives, and pain killers. When you visit your doctor, take along the list of drugs you are taking. This way, there will be no confusion or mistakes about the high blood pressure drugs or other drugs you are using.

Keep a list of any over-the-counter drugs you regularly take.

DRUGS FOR HYPERTENSION

Blood pressure drugs can be divided into several types. Following are some of the types of medications available. Please see the chart for more detailed information.

Alpha Blockers

These medications reduce nerve impulses to blood vessels. Blood is then able to pass more easily through the vessels causing the blood pressure to go down. Examples of these drugs are Cardura® (doxazosin mesylate) and Hytrin® (terazosin hydrochloride) among others.

Alpha blockers are mostly used as add-on drugs, rather than for the first drug therapy, in treating hypertension. These drugs have been very useful in men with urinary symptoms related to prostate enlargement, even when hypertension was not present. A potential side effect of these drugs is that sometimes, when a rapid upright position is taken, blood pressure falls to a greater degree than normal. This overly steep fall in blood pressure may be associated with dizziness in some patients. These drugs also have been linked to extreme tiredness. Alpha blockers do, however, work well as blood pressure medications.

Angiotensin Converting Enzyme Inhibitors

ACE inhibitors are drugs that in the end lower the blood pressure by causing the blood vessels to relax and open wider.

ACE inhibitors have also proven useful in protecting the kidney in persons with reduced kidney function and appear to protect persons with diabetes from having further problems such as kidney failure, heart failure, and heart attack, all to a degree greater than expected.

While this class of drugs has long been thought to be less effective in African Americans, a recent study showed that the ACE inhibitor ramipril did lower blood pressure in African Americans with reduced kidney function when taken with other antihypertensive drugs.

If you have diabetes, reduced kidney function and/or heart

ORAL ANTIHYPERTENSIVE DRUGS AND THEIR SIDE-EFFECTS

Drug	Trade Name	Usual Dose Range, Total mg/day* (Frequency per Day)	Selected Side Effects and Comments*
DIURETICS (PARTIAL LIST)			
			Short-term: increase cholesterol and glucose levels; biochemical abnormalities: decreases potassium, sodium, and magnesium levels, increases uric acid and calcium levels; rare: blood dyscrasias, photosensitivity, pancreatitis, hyponatremia
Chlorthalidone (G)†	Hygroton®	12.5–50 (1)	
Hydrochlorothiazide (G)	Hydrodiuril, Esidrix®	12.5–50 (1)	
Indapamide	Lozol®	1.25–5 (1)	(Less or no hypercholesterolemia)
Metrolazone	Mykrox®	0.5–1.0 (1)	
	Zaroxolyn®	2.5–10 (1)	
Loop diuretics			
Bumetanide (G)	Bumex®	0.5–4 (2–3)	(Short duration of action, no hypercalcemia)
Ethacrynic acid	Edecrin®	25–100 (2–3)	Only nonsulfonamide diuretic, ototoxicity)
Furosemide (G)	Lasix®	40–240 (2–3)	(Short duration of action, no hypercalcemia)
Torsemide	Demadex®	5–100 (1–2)	
Potassium-sparing agents			
Amiloride hydrochloride (G)	Midamor®	5–10 (1)	
Spironolactone (G)	Aldactone®	25–100 (1)	(Gynecomastia)
Triamterene (G)	Dyrenium®	25–200 (1)	
ADRENERGIC INHIBITORS			
Peripheral agents			
Guanadrel	Hylorel®	10–75 (2)	(Postural hypotension, diarrhea)
Guanethidine monosulfate	Ismelin®	10–150 (1)	(Postural hypotension, diarrhea)

Drug	Trade Name	Usual Dose Range, Total mg/day[*] (Frequency per Day)	Selected Side Effects and Comments[*]
Reserpine (G)[**]	Serpasil®	0.05–0.25 (1)	(Nasal congestion, sedation, depression, activation of peptic ulcer) Sedation, dry mouth, brady-cardia, withdrawal hypertension
Central alpha-agonists			
Clonidine hydrochloride (G)	Catapres®	0.2–1.2 (2–3)	(More withdrawal)
Guanabenz acetate (G)	Wytensin®	8–32 (2)	
Guanfacine hydrochloride (G)	Tenex®	1–3 (1)	(Less withdrawal)
Methyldopa (G)	Aldomet®	500–3,000 (2)	(Hepatic and "autoimmune" disorders)
Alpha-blockers			
Doxazosin mesylate	Cardura®	1–16 (1)	
Prazosin hydrochloride (G)	Minipress®	2–30 (2–3)	
Terazosin hydrochloride	Hytrin®	1–20 (1)	
Beta-blockers			Bronchospasm, bradycardia, heart failure, may mask insulin-induced hypoglycemia; less serious: impaired peripheral circulation, insomnia, fatigue, decreased exercise tolerance, hypertriglyceridemia (except agents with intrinsic sympathomimetric activity)
Acebutolol§‡	Sectral®	200–800 (1)	
Atenolol (G)§	Tenormi®n	25–100 (1–2)	
Betaxolol§	Kerlone®	5–20 (1)	
Bisoprolol fumarate§	Zebeta®	2.5–10 (1)	
Carteolol hydrochloride‡	Cartrol®	2.5–10 (1)	
Metoprolol tartrate (G)§	Lopresso®r	50–300 (2)	
Metoprolol succinate§	Toprol-XL®	50–300 (1)	
Nadolol (G)	Corgard®	40–320 (1)	
Penbutolol sulfate‡	Levatol®	10–20 (1)	
Pindolol (G)‡	Visken®	10–60 (2)	

Drugs for Hypertension

Drug	Trade Name	Usual Dose Range, Total mg/day* (Frequency per Day)	Selected Side Effects and Comments*
Propranolol hydrochloride (G)	Inderal® Inderal LA®	40–480 (1) 40–480 (2	
Timolol maleate (G)	Blocadren®	20–60 (2)	
Combined alpha- and beta-blockers			Postural hypotension, bronchospasm
Carvedilol	Coreg®	12.5–50 (2)	
Labetalol hydrochloride (G)	Normodyne®, Trandate®	200–1,200 (2)	

DIRECT VASODILATORS

Drug	Trade Name	Dose	Comments
Hydralazine hydrochloride (G)	Apresoline®	50–300 (2)	(Lupus syndrome)
Minoxidil (G)	Loniten®	5–100 (1)	(Hirsutism)

CALCIUM ANTAGONISTS

Nondihydropyridines

Drug	Trade Name	Dose	Comments
Diltiazem hydrochloride	Cardizem SR®	120–360 (2)	(Nausea, headache)
	Cardizem CD®	120–360 (1)	
	Dilacor XR®, Tiazac®		
Mibefradil dihydrochloride (T-channel calcium antagonist)		50–100 (1)	(No worsening of systolic dysfunction,' contraindicated with terfenadine [Seldane], astemizole [Hismanal], and cisapride
Verapamil hydrochloride	Isoptin SR,® Calan SR	90–480 (2)	(Constipation)
	Verelan®, Covera HS	120–480 (1)	

Dihydropyridines			Edema of the ankle, flushing, headache
Amlodipine besylate	Norvasc®	2.5–10 (1)	
Felodipine	Plendil®	2.5–20 (1)	
Isradipine	DynaCirc®	5–20 (2)	
	DynaCirc CR®	5–20 (1)	
Nicardipine	Cardene SR®	60–90 (2)	

Drug	Trade Name	Usual Dose Range, Total mg/day* (Frequency per Day)	Selected Side Effects and Comments*
Nifedipine	Procardia XL® Adalat CC®	30–120 (1)	
Nisoldipine	Sular®	20–60 (1)	

ACE INHIBITORS

			Common: cough; rare: angioedema, hyperkalemia, rash, loss of taste, leukopenia
Benazerpril hydrochloride	Lotensin®	5–40 (1–2)	
Captopril (G)	Capoten®	25–150 (2–3)	
Enalapril maleate	Vasotec®	5–40 (1–2)	
Fosinopril sodium	Monopril®	10–40 (1–2)	
Lisinopril	Prinivil®, Zestril®	5–40 (1)	
Moexipril	Univasc®	7.5–15 (2)	
Quinarpil hydrochloride	Accupril®	5–80 (1–2)	
Ramipril	Altace®	1.25–20 (1–2)	
Trandolapril	Mavik®	1–4 (1)	

ANGIOTENSIN II RECEPTOR BLOCKERS

			Angioedema (very rare), hyperkalemia
Losartan potassium	Cozaar®	25–100 (1–2)	
Valsartan	Diovan®	80–320 (1)	
Irbesartan	Avapro®	150–300 (1)	

* These dosages may vary from those listed in the Physicians' Desk Reference (51st edition), which may be consulted for additional information. The listing of side effects is not all-inclusive, and side effects are for the class of drugs where noted for individual drugs (in parenthesis); clinicians are urged to refer to the package insert for a more detailed listing.
† (G) indicated generic available.
‡ Has iintrinsic sympathomimetic activity.
§ Cardioselective.
** Also acts centrally.

Reprinted from JNC VI.

failure, ACE inhibitors can help you. Drugs in this class include Capoten® (captopril), Lotensin® (benazerpril hydrochloride), Monopril® (fosinopril sodium) and others.

The most common side effect of ACE inhibitors is a dry cough. In some patients ACE inhibitors may cause a rise in serum creatinine (an indicator of kidney function) and/or serum potassium. In most cases, however, the ACE inhibitor will not need to be stopped.

A more serious, though infrequent, side effect of ACE inhibitors is a swelling of the skin, lips, tongue, throat, or in severe cases, the airways in the lung (called angioedema). Patients who get these symptoms in most instances should have their ACE inhibitor stopped. Your doctor will probably monitor your kidneys and watch your blood pressure closely if you are taking an ACE inhibitor.

Angiotensin II Antagonists/Receptor Blockers (ACE IIs/ARBs)

These medications protect the blood vessels from a hormone called angiotensin II. The drugs cause the blood vessels to become wider and therefore the blood pressure goes down.

Angiotensin receptor blockers are fairly new antihypertensive drugs. They are often used together with water pills to treat high blood pressure. In general, over the long term, angiotensin receptor blockers are thought to be better tolerated by patients than are ACEs. That is, patients who take these drugs stop taking them less often than other drugs.

Though ACE IIs/ARBs have similarities to the ACE inhibitors, patients generally do not cough with these drugs. Although ankle and facial swelling can occur when using ACE

IIs/ARBs, it's less common than with the ACE inhibitors. Several recent studies have found that angiotensin receptor blockers prevent kidney disease complications better in people with diabetes than other drugs. Nevertheless, angiotensin receptor blockers usually need to be prescribed along with other drugs to control blood pressure in people with diabetes and/or reduced kidney function.

This class includes Avapro® (irbesartan), Cozaar® (losartum potassium) and others.

Adrenergic Inhibitors

These drugs reduce the activity of the sympathetic nervous system and, similar to the beta blockers and some calcium antagonists, may slow the heart rate. These drugs are not usually prescribed as the first drug treatment for hypertension. Though these drugs do lower blood pressure, they usually cause more side effects than other antihypertensive drug classes. Adrenergic inhibitors tend to be less well tolerated by patients over the long-term.

Typical side effects of adrenergic inhibitors include dry mouth and sedation. These drugs should not generally be prescribed or taken at the same time as beta blockers. Also, if a patient abruptly stops taking these drugs it can lead to a risc in blood pressure. Adrenergic inhibitors are most often used as add-on treatment when blood pressure has not been controlled with more commonly used drugs.

Beta Blockers

Your doctor may prescribe a beta blocker, also known as a beta adrenergic receptor blocker.

This drug makes the heart beat slower and with less force,

which helps blood pressure go down. It does this by reducing the nerve impulses to the heart and the blood vessels.

Beta blockers are often used together with diuretics to lower blood pressure. Beta blockers are the drugs of choice in people who have survived a heart attack and also are very useful in those with heart failure.

Beta blockers are very effective in lowering blood pressure. A few common beta blockers are Sectral® (acebutolol), Tenormin® (atenolol), Kerlone® (betaxolol), Levatol® (penbutolol sulfate) and Lopressor® (metoprolol tartrate). Beta blockers can, in some cases, cause sleeplessness, spasms in the lungs similar to asthma, and heart failure. You should avoid beta blockers if you have asthma or reactive airways disease because they can narrow the airways and cause wheezing as well as shortness of breath. Beta blockers can sometimes cause impotence in men, though not as much as seen with diuretics.

Abruptly stopping any beta blocker can lead to a very large rise in blood pressure and a greater risk of heart attack. If your doctor prescribes beta blockers for you, he or she will want to watch and check your heart and lungs closely. If you have asthma your doctor may prescribe a different drug.

Calcium Channel Blockers/Calcium Antagonists

These medications stop calcium from entering the muscle cells of the heart and blood vessels. This action causes blood vessels to relax and open wider and, therefore, lowers the blood pressure.

Calcium channel blockers include Norvasc® (amlodipine besylate), Cardizem® and Dilacor® (diltiazem hydrochloride), and Verlan® (verapamil hydrochloride). Some possible side effects of calcium channel blockers may include headache, flushing, leg swelling and dizziness. Certain calcium channel blockers, such as Cardizem®, Dilacor®, and Verlan®, should not be taken with allergy medicines as they may cause nausea, constipation, and a slow heart rate.

Calcium antagonists are commonly used high blood pressure medications that work well. They are often used together with ACE inhibitors and ARBs in persons with diabetes and/or reduced kidney function.

A possible side effect of the calcium antagonists is swelling of the lower legs. If calcium channel blockers are taken together with ACE inhibitors, this swelling will decrease. In summary, calcium antagonists are safe and highly effective blood pressure lowering medications.

Direct Vasodilators

These agents are used less often than most other antihypertensive drug classes. They cause the blood vessels to relax but they do so directly. They relax the muscle in the wall of blood vessels, and so open the blood vessels, which makes blood pressure come down. These drugs are usually prescribed when other drugs have been tried. Examples of direct vasodilators include minoxidil and hydralazine.

Because these drugs usually cause people to retain salt and water in their bodies, you should, at the same time you take them, also take a powerful diuretic. Also, either a calcium antagonist or a beta blocker is often necessary to slow the rise in heart rate that can sometimes occur. These drugs include Apresoline® (hydralazine hydrochloride), Loniten® (minoxidil) and others.

One potential side effect to watch for is that hydralazine may cause symptoms similar to lupus, an immune disorder. These drugs also may cause a loss of appetite, stomach aches,

Diuretics

One of the most common types of blood pressure medications are diuretics. They help your kidneys clear excess fluid and sodium from your body, so they will cause you to urinate more. They are also known as "water pills." The excess fluid may be part of the reason that your blood pressure is high.

Diuretics usually begin lowering blood pressure within weeks. When you are given a diuretic, your doctor may want you to return for a blood pressure check-up in a few weeks to see if the drug is working.

Diuretics can lower blood pressure very well when taken alone. If you take more than two antihypertensive drugs in most cases at least one of them should be a diuretic. In men, diuretics are more likely than any other drug to cause impotence. Another side effect of these drugs may be low serum potassium. The risk of having low potassium when using diuretics can be greatly reduced by cutting back on the salt in your diet. So try to eat less of it.

Diuretics have a few side effects. You may lose potassium and magnesium, two necessary minerals, along with the water you excrete, or lose, daily. To counteract this, your doctor may prescribe potassium pills for you. Diuretics can upset the way your body uses, or metabolizes, glucose, the simple sugar the body needs for energy. Diuretics also may increase the amount of cholesterol in your blood. The doctor will check for these problems if you are taking a diuretic.

PATIENT RESPONSIBILITIES

Good treatment depends on being able to openly and freely talk to your doctor. As a patient, you must expect the best of your physicians and other health care providers who treat your high blood pressure. You should be sure that

- you have open, two-way communication

- you are told and educated about hypertension

- you are treated fairly and with dignity and respect when you call or visit your doctor

At the same time, you, the patient, must help your physicians get your blood pressure under control. You can help your blood pressure and take fewer medications to control blood pressure if you adopt good dietary and lifestyle habits. Also, you must know what your goal blood pressure should be. And, if you have not gotten to a lower blood pressure over a reasonable period of time, you must ask your physician what his/her plans are for getting you to that goal.

Be patient. Know that it takes many weeks for blood pressure lowering drugs to fully work. But they do work, so don't stop taking your pills without talking to your doctor. The faster your blood pressure falls, the more likely you are to feel bad; however, this bad feeling almost always sorts itself out after a short period of time. Work with your physician and his/her nurses and other staff to clearly understand what medicines you should take and how often you

Realize that it takes many weeks for blood pressure lowering drugs to fully work.

are to take them. Do not make changes in the way you take your medication without talking to your physician. Finally, when you reach your target blood pressure level, feel good that the joint efforts of you and your doctor have paid off. You've beaten the odds! If you don't reach your goals, don't worry. Many patients with hypertension who take blood pressure lowering medications do not reach their goal but do control their high blood pressure through diet, exercise, and medication. They are all important.

IN A NUTSHELL

- If your doctor prescribes blood pressure medicine, take it regularly as prescribed, even if you are feeling great.

- You can best remember to take your pills if you take them at the same time each day and always keep them in the same place.

- Your pharmacist can give you information sheets for the drugs you use. The pharmacist will also be glad to answer your questions about these drugs.

- Medication for hypertension may make you feel bad for a brief time when you begin to take it, but in the long run, it will make you feel much better.

In A Nutshell, *continued*

- As a patient, you have the right to expect your doctor to treat you fairly, with dignity and respect, and to talk to you openly. Your doctor should explain your illness to you in a way you can understand.

- You must follow the treatment program your doctor gives because you wish to take an active part in getting healthy again. Always understand why your doctor has prescribed the treatment he or she has.

CHAPTER SIX

Healthy Eating and Lifestyle

Your doctor has told you that your blood pressure is high. Let this be, for you, a clear call to change one part of your life and to begin another. Yes, it causes pain to know we must give up what we are used to. But it also causes joy to make changes that we know are for the better. In this chapter we will show you the way to that joy.

Your doctor may have prescribed medication for you. He probably also has said you must change your diet, begin exercising, quit smoking, and slow down if you want to get well. Yes, this may look like a tall order, and you may feel burdened. Yet the drill is simple. To make hard, long-term changes you must first look inward, telling yourself again why the changes are so important, and remembering that you owe it to yourself and your loved ones to take the best care you can of your health and well-being.

Second, start small. Maybe you need to tell yourself, this first week I'll get into a routine with my medicine. Next week, I'll sign up at the gym and start that exercise class I've been thinking about, or start taking daily walks with my friends. In the third week, when I have these things in place, I can start learning how to cook healthier food for myself and my family.

Patience and resolve have gotten many others to good health. What they have done, you can too.

Remind yourself that people feel better when they eat well, are a healthy weight, and exercise. Ask them! Seek out friends who are taking care of themselves. They'll have heartening stories to tell you. They'll help you see that knowing you have hypertension is an open door to a new and better way of living, an invitation to be more relaxed, enjoy more energy, and live longer.

Again, the key to making these changes is to go slowly and take it step by step. Maybe when you begin to exercise you can only get to the corner and back. Fine, do that for a week and you'll find that you're ready to walk around the block. Before long, a half hour walk each day will seem easy. You'll look forward to it. You'll enjoy the fresh air, you'll look at the flowers, and you'll begin to feel a new strength in your body that will make you smile with pleasure.

Try eating one extra piece of fruit a day.

Or, let's say your doctor tells you to eat foods with potassium, like fresh fruit. Try eating one extra piece of fruit a day. Do this for a few weeks. Soon, it will feel normal, as if it has always been part of your regular diet. Then add another piece of fruit or juice and so on, until you reach your target.

Before you begin making any changes in your lifestyle, check in with your doctor, nurse, or dietician so you know exactly what you are to do: the foods you are to eat, the total calories, the amount of salt you are allowed. Make sure you know what type of exercise you should do, and for how long and how many times each week.

BEING READY FOR CHANGE

You will only begin to make a change when you are ready. Readiness is a state of mind that determines how we move towards making decisions about changing the way we act in our everyday lives.

> *You will only begin to make a change when you are ready.*

   Not being ready means you haven't yet thought about making the change, or you don't see how changing will do you any good. *But if you've read this far, you **are** ready.* You know why the changes are so important. Just knowing that means you have already begun to change. At the other end of the line is the person who is now fully ready to make a change.

   As a person who is ready, you'll face change with greater strength. Sure, you may at first meet some resistance from within. You want to exercise but you just can't get started. Maybe you tell yourself, "Well, I'll start next week or maybe next month when things calm down," or "As soon as I get enough money to buy a stationary bike, then I'll start exercising," or "As soon as the weather gets better, then I'll start," or "My back hurts today, maybe tomorrow I'll feel better." No. Understand that in the beginning of something new you'll meet all kinds of internal resistance. Know it for what it is, a kind of static place. Then argue back and simply say to yourself, "Well, excuse me, but I'm starting now. I'm ready."

HOW TO MAKE CHANGES

Even after you begin, days will come when you will ask yourself, "Why aren't I eating my favorite foods anymore?" and "Why am I getting up every morning to take a walk?" You know the answer. You are doing it because it's good for you. How it's good is different for everyone. Some people tell us, "I need to live to see my grandchildren grow up." Others say, "I love my job. It would be terrible for me if I got too sick to work." Some people just want to set a good example for their children. Others want to look good even as they grow older. And for some, it's simply a matter of stubborn independence, "I just don't want to have to rely on anyone to take care of me as long as I can take care of myself." Find the benefit that means the most to you, and keep reminding yourself of it as a way of pushing yourself on.

Sure, in the beginning you may lack confidence, or even courage. Maybe you've been telling yourself for too long, "I don't have what it takes" to do this or to do that. Or, "I've never made a deliberate change in my life. How can I start now?" Sometimes, we, as doctors, hear these people say, "No matter how hard I try, I can't seem to get my blood pressure under control." One patient, a middle aged mother, grumbled, "How can I eat the right things when my family wants me to fix the foods I'm not supposed to eat?" Finally, a male patient of about forty-five, said when we recommended exercise, "I only know of one person who has started walking and kept it up. So what's the point of starting?"

This is a hurdle that you can get over. There's a voice in all of us that makes a lot of noise when we let it. Little by little we can develop the positive will that will silence that voice. You can begin to build confidence by starting small. Each little success makes you more ready for the bigger ones. That's why exercise is so wonderful. You can start wherever you are, and if you keep it up, you'll see progress. Soon, you'll feel it too, in the new pleasure you'll get from your body.

The key is to take the first step. Courage and confidence then follows. We all know doubt, shame, and fear. They don't matter. Go forward anyway. Take the first step. And when you fall, and you will, get back up and move forward.

> *The key is to take the first step.*

EXERCISE AND WEIGHT CONTROL

Exercise is one of the keys to staying healthy, yet many Americans do not get exercise at all. The figures tells us that 40 percent of adults had no leisure-time physical activity and only 15 percent spent thirty minutes a day in moderate physical activity, like walking. Worse, Blacks are usually less physically active than whites. According to American Heart Association statistics, just a shade under 50 percent of non-Hispanic Blacks are "sedentary"—that is, they get no exercise at all. People who are sedentary are more likely to get a disease. One of the diseases they are especially apt to get is hypertension.

One of the aims of this book is to change this statistic. To a large part you can do this by making a series of individual choices. The choice to stay as healthy as you can be is very important. It's a way of respecting our reality *and honoring the power that created us.*

All this can start when you decide to begin exercising.

Remember, obesity is bad for your health, and the end product of being sedentary is getting fat. Scientists have technical ways of measuring obesity, but most of us don't need a formula. We see it all around us, and maybe in the mirror. Indeed, obesity has become so great a danger that former Surgeon General David Satcher thinks it may "soon cause as much preventable disease and death as cigarette smoking," and proposed community action programs to address it.

We take Dr. Satcher's ideas most seriously. We agree also with the strong words of Health and Human Services Secretary Tommy G. Thompson, who said:

> Our modern environment has allowed these conditions to increase at alarming rates and become a growing health problem for our nation. By confronting these conditions, we have tremendous opportunities to prevent the unnecessary disease and disability they portend for our future.

There is cause to worry that from 1991 to 2000, obesity among American adults increased 61 percent. And, once again, the increase has been far more dramatic among Blacks and Hispanics than among whites.

Yes, these are national and community problems and their final solution must be worked on politically, in communities. But in the meantime, there is much you can do for yourself.

WHY YOU DON'T EXERCISE

The surveys tell us that sedentary people give a number of reasons for not exercising.

1. Exercise is stressful and I get enough stress at work.

2. Rest is more important than exercise.

3. Weight training may hurt me or injure me.

4. Exercise is bad for the heart.

5. My neighborhood is dangerous so I can't walk.

6. I prefer exercising in a group but I don't know of any near me.

7. I don't have the time or money to join a YMCA or club.

8. I don't have anyone to watch my kids while I exercise.

9. I have too many other duties already.

10. I'm too old and too out of shape.

11. My hair will get messed up.

12. The damage is already done, I'll just take medication.

You may see yourself in one or several of the answers. Some of the answers are obviously untrue. People who exercise regularly find it the opposite of stressful. It allows them to unwind. Rest and exercise are both important to your health. Exercise, according to your age and condition, is good for the heart.

Others are pretty thin excuses. Sure, your neighborhood may be bad, but you can probably get to a nearby mall or park where you can do your morning walks. Yes, weight training *can* harm you, but not if you learn what you are doing in a good exercise program, and not as long as you don't overdo it. Babysitting can be a problem, but if worse comes to worst, put the baby in a stroller and make that walk with her your exercise.

About messing up your hair, you've gotta be kidding. You're going to look us in the eye and say you'd rather mess up your heart than your hair? C'mon.

FINDING A PROGRAM

To the experts, a good exercise program means moderate or intense physical activity for thirty minutes at least three times a week. How you do that depends on your condition and your taste. The almost endless list of ways to exercise includes

- running

- dancing

- brisk walking

- swimming

- playing basketball

- playing tennis

- doing aerobics

Programs for all of these are run at your local Y or fitness club, and there are probably many local agencies nearby that run exercise programs. You can surely find one if you look around. Such groups have the benefit of teaching and energizing you, and giving you the pleasure of exercising with others doing the same thing. For many people, the place they exercise becomes a real club, where long-lasting friendships are made.

a good exercise program means moderate or strenuous physical activity for thirty minutes at least three times a week.

If you choose dancing or a team sport, once again, the benefit will be both physical and social.

We realize that not everyone can enjoy the pleasures of group exercise. If for whatever reason that road isn't open for you, you can work out in your home. Go to a video shop or the public library, and get one of the many workout tapes on the market. Look them over and see what suits you best. Or get up early and exercise along with the exercise programs on many local television stations.

Whatever you do, remember, start slowly, let your body feel its way back toward good health. Whatever you do, talk it over with your doctor. Between you, decide what kind of exercise program will best suit your needs, your condition, and your taste.

In the beginning, you might go for a fifteen-minute work-out three times a week. If, for whatever reason, that seems to be too much, you could start just doing five minutes—say, a walk around the block. You'll find that you'll be able gradually to build that time up, with your goal as thirty minutes three times a week.

HOW MANY CALORIES ARE YOU BURNING?

Activity	Total Calories/hour
Walking slowly (2.5 mph)	210-230
Brisk walking (4.0 mph)	250-345
Jogging (6 mph)	315-480
Cycling	315-480
Basketball	480-625
Swimming	480-625

Walking is ideal exercise. It requires a little equipment but not much: good walking shoes and clothing that makes sense for the kind of weather it is. People who get into the walking habit enjoy walking in all kinds of weather. Just dress warmly enough when it's cold, dry enough when it's wet. And, of course, if you're walking in winter conditions, be very careful not to slip.

Some people prefer indoor walking. Malls are excellent places for this; more and more churches are urging parishioners to do their exercise there, by walking around the church.

The beauty of exercise is that the payoffs come quickly. Before long, you'll find that you're sleeping better, have more energy, and enjoy your meals more. It's amazing!

Once you get "hooked" on exercise, you may find other ways to stretch your legs. Instead of driving to the grocery store you might want to walk and carry a few bags home—which is great exercise for the legs and upper body. At work, you might choose to park at the far end of the parking lot, or take the subway and walk a few extra blocks. Or you might find yourself taking the stairs instead of the elevator. You'll do that because it makes you feel good.

The fact that so many people get little or no exercise is built into our culture. Cars help make us that way. So do computers and television. And obesity is built in too, with fast food calling out to us from every street corner. So we move less and eat more fat and other foods that are bad for us.

A BALANCED DIET

The American Heart Association recommends that no more than 30 percent of your total daily calories should come from fat. That's about 67 grams. If you go to Burger King and eat a double whopper with cheese, that's your 67 grams of fat right there. Imagine how those grams add up when you also go nibbling through the day.

No, we're not on an anti-eating campaign. Eating is one of the joys of life. (See the chart on page 94 for a list of some common snacks and their "nutritional" contents.)

A healthy balanced diet includes

- hearty breads and cereals (with a variety of grains)

- low-fat, high-protein meals like fish and skinless chicken

- fresh fruits and fresh green vegetables

FAT, CHOLESTEROL, CALORIES, AND SODIUM CONTENT IN JUNK FOODS

Snack (1 ounce)	Saturated Fat (grams)	Cholesterol (mgs)	Total Fat (grams)	Calories from Fat (%)	Total Calories	Sodium (mgs)
Pretzels, salted (1 oz. is about 5 twists, 3 1/4 x 2 1/4 x 1/4 in.)	0.2	0	1.0	8	108	486
Popcorn, air popped without salt (1 oz. is about 3 1/2 cups)	0.2	0	1.2	10	108	1
Tortilla chips, lower fat (light) nacho flavor	0.8	1	4.3	31	126	284
Corn Chips	1.3	0	9.5	56	153	179
Popcorn, popped with oil and salt (1 oz. is about 2 1/2 cups)	1.4	0	8.0	51	142	251
Tortilla chips, nacho flavor	1.4	1	7.3	47	141	201
Trail mix (1 oz. is about 1/5 cups	1.6	0	8.3	57	131	65
Potato chips	3.1	0	9.8	58	152	168

Reprinted from NIHLBI, "Step by Step: Eating to Lower Your Blood Cholesterol" (February 1999), p. 10.

Also, cutting down on fats, sugar, and fried foods will do you a world of good.

A balanced diet gives you more energy, helps keep you healthy, and adds years to your life. As good as such a diet is, it is especially good for a person with high blood pressure and heart disease. Eating foods high in fats and cholesterol, including soul food cooked in the old-fashioned way, is bad for you. Yes, soul food as we know it is not good for high blood pressure or for your heart. Try it without lard or butter or fatty meat and without high salt. Otherwise, limit these foods to special times, like Christmas, Thanksgiving, or your birthday. It is rich food!

If you have high blood pressure and are sensitive to salt your doctor has probably advised you to cut way back on salt. We go a bit further in this chapter. We talk about how to eat a low-salt diet but also how to eat a healthier diet overall. For some people, eating a low-salt diet will help keep blood pressure under control. Eating a low-fat diet rich in vitamins and minerals may help you to avoid heart disease, especially if you exercise. (For more on diet, see *The Black Man's Guide to Good Health: Essential Advice for African American Men and Their Families,* by James W. Reed, M.D., Neil Shulman, M.D., and Charlene Shucker.; *The Heart of the Matter: The African American's Guide to Heart Disease, Heart Treatment, and Heart Wellness,* by Hilton M. Hudson, II, M.D. and Herbert Stern, Ph.D.; and *Weight Loss for African American Women: 8 Weeks to Better Health,* by George Edmond Smith, M.D., all available from Hilton Publishing Company. Visit Hilton's website, www.hiltonpub.com for free recipes.).

You may also enjoy the foods that some call typical soul

foods: Foods such as salty collard greens, smoked pork, ribs, fried chicken, and macaroni and cheese.

Unfortunately, these foods, made like our grandparents made them, are usually high in fat and calories. They're bad for us. It's a pain just thinking about turning away from food that's fed the body and the soul down the years. But the bitter truth is that eating this food is making us heartsick. It is killing us.

Now the good news. You don't have to give up soul food; just learn to like it with less frying, less fat, and less salt. You should also stay away from junk food and fast food, which as we've explained, causes all sorts of trouble.

Let the truth energize you. If our diets are high in fat, obesity, hypertension, and heart disease will probably result.

We think you can do what you have to, especially when you discover, as you will later in this chapter, that you can still eat delicious food that tastes like your mother's, but is healthier for you.

WEIGHT LOSS

You may want to lose weight and start on a diet. Before you do, tell your doctor and ask for his or her advice. If you have health insurance, you may be able to talk to a dietician as part of your covered health plan. Your doctor will probably tell you to slowly reduce the amount of calories you are eating, while getting exercise too. This way, you are more likely to stick with the diet as a way of life and to stay at a good weight. If you blow your diet one day, one week, or one month, forgive yourself and get back on track. Don't quit on yourself.

Quickie diets or crash diets are useless. They don't keep weight off, and some of them are just plain bad for your health. Doing drastic diets, and then going on and off different diets, can be punishing to your body and may be dangerous to the heart. We urge you to stay away from crash diets and, instead, to seek out good eating habits of the kind we outline here. These are habits that you can keep all your life and share with your family. That's one way we can make obesity and hypertension less of a community and nation-wide health threat than it is.

> *Avoid crash diets and, instead, seek out good eating habits.*

One last suggestion before we get down to some nuts and bolts: If you're trying to stay on a healthy diet and to lose weight, we recommend that you keep a diet log, listing each day what and when you eat. You might also want to include a line about your mood. Overeating can sometimes be caused by boredom, stress or loneliness, frustration or anxiety. As you become more aware of your mood, you might be better able to control the urge to make yourself feel good by eating what you don't need. The sad fact is that method doesn't work. (On page 173 of Dr. George Edmond Smith's *Weight Loss for African American Women,* you'll find a list of questions to help you learn whether or not you have an eating disorder, and, if so, how bad it is.)

Looking at your diet log, you can see if you are getting too many calories from snacks and fast food. Your doctor or dietician can give you a chart of foods with calories noted that will make your logging simpler and more exact. Your doctor can also give you information on vitamins, minerals, and protein, and you may want to monitor your intake of these too in your log.

DASH DIET

In 1997 the *New England Journal of Medicine* published a study called "Dietary Approaches to Stop Hypertension," known as DASH. The study found that a low-fat diet high in fiber, fruits and vegetables, greatly helped lower blood pressure in people of all races. But, strikingly, the benefit of such a diet was twice as great in African Americans.

The DASH diet proved to lower blood pressure just as well as some blood pressure medications did. That's why the diet is recommended by the National Heart Lung and Blood Institute. The diet reduces calories, fat, cholesterol and sodium. At the same time, it encourages you to eat fruits, vegetables, low fat dairy foods, and to avoid saturated fats. It also recommends the use of whole grains, poultry, fish, and nuts.

This diet, along with other lifestyle changes and, when needed, medications, has been shown to be an effective way to lower blood pressure. Your doctor can give you more information on DASH. You can also find out more by consulting the website:www.discoverfitness.com/The_DASH_Diet.html; or by calling 800-575-WELL.

Some of the items suggested in the DASH diet may be new for you and your family, so phase in these new meals over time. Before long, you and your family may find that your eating habits have changed for the good without anybody going into shock.

While your doctor can tell you how many calories are right for you, the general DASH plan is based on 2,000 calories a day. The number of daily servings in a food group may vary from those listed based on your own caloric needs

SALT

If you have high blood pressure and are sensitive to salt, it's very important that you cut back on the amount of salt you eat. Perhaps you will choose to change your whole diet and to begin the DASH or other program. But if you are not ready for that, you still should make one change in your diet, and that is to cut way back on salt.

Remember that adults should eat no more than 3,000 milligrams (mgs) of salt per day. But American food makers love salt, it is in almost everything, so most Americans eat far more than 3,000–4,000 mgs per day. Your doctor may ask you to eat as little as 500 mgs per day. If you want to reduce the amount of salt you eat each day, you will have to be very, very careful about which foods you choose to eat.

Junk foods, fast foods, prepared foods, and even many ready-to-eat cakes and cookies, are high in salt. As an example, eating a Burger King Double Whopper with cheese provides 1,460 mgs of salt, or more than half your daily allowance. If you add fries, you are over 3,000 mgs. If you eat a dessert, you will be way above 3,000! The same is true of fast food fried chicken. It tastes so good because of the high level of salt in the "secret recipe" bread coating. Not to mention the gobs of saturated fat and high amount of calories.

The people who design fast food menus don't aim to make

DAILY FOOD RECOMMENDATIONS

Food Group	Daily Servings (except as noted)	Serving Sizes
Grains & grain products	5-12	1 slice bread 1 cup ready-to-eat cereal* cup cooked rice, pasta, or cereal
Vegetables	3-5	1 cup raw leafy vegetable cup cooked vegetable 6 ounces vegetable juice
Fruits	2-4	1 medium fruit cup dried fruit cup fresh, frozen, or canned fruit 6 ounces fruit juice
Lowfat or fat free dairy foods	2-3	8 ounces milk 1 cup yogurt 1 ounce cheese
Lean meats, poultry, and fish	3 or less	3 ounces cooked lean meats, skinless poultry, or fish
Nuts, seeds, and dry beans	4-5 per week	1/3 cup or 1 ounce nuts 1 tablespoon or 1 ounce seeds cup cooked dry beans
*Fats & oils***	moderation	1 teaspoon soft margarine 1 tablespoon low fat mayonnaise 2 tablespoons light salad dressing 1 teaspoon vegetable oil
Sweets	use sparingly	1 tablespoon sugar 1 tablespoon jelly or jam ounce jelly beans 8 ounces lemonade

* Serving sizes vary. Check the product's nutrition label.
** Fat content changes. Check the label carefully to determine how much fat is in the food and oil you use.

them healthy. They aim to make them taste good, which often is *not* the same thing. Remember, their goal is profit. Yours is good health. Fast food restaurants advertise heavily, often aiming their ads at children, and often aiming them at African Americans. But you don't have to play their game. You have a better game of your own. The next time you feel the need to eat fast foods, remember that while they seem like a tasty bargain, these foods can rob you of your health.

> *The people who design fast food menus don't aim to make them healthy. They aim to make them taste good, which often is not the same thing.*

At first you may find it hard to give up salty foods in general. But you may change your mind. If you stay away from fast foods and other salty foods for two months, then treat yourself to a big fried chicken meal, you may find it doesn't taste as good any more. Your taste buds will have changed, and too much salt will shock your tongue and taste buds.

Ask people on a low-salt diet, and they will tell you about this change in taste. They will also tell you that they enjoy the new range of herbs and spices that they've started to use instead of salt.

HOW TO CUT BACK ON SALT

A good first step to cutting back the amount of salt in your diet is to stop adding table salt to your food and in your cooking. Keep in mind that there is also high salt in soy sauce, in ready-made salad dressings, and in many hot and spicy seasonings. You can easily lower your salt intake and have better tasting food by making your own dressings and choosing and adding your own spices. Maybe you'll like some hot peppers (just a bit) for added zest. Basil and oregano have strong flavors that people like. Little by little your taste buds will adjust to less salt and you will begin to taste all those other flavors you have been missing!

If you have a favorite food that you just can't stand doing without, such as a favorite bread for toast in the morning, try eating less of it. Eat just one slice of the favorite and one slice of a lower salt bread so you'll stay within the limit of the daily amount of sodium you should have. Over time, you may be able to give up even that favorite, but too salty, food.

If you cut down on salt in your cooking, stay away from salty ready-made food and fast foods, you'll soon reach the goal you want, the one you've set with your doctor.

Read food labels. They tell you how much salt is in any ready-made food you buy. You may be surprised to find that just one or two portions of many foods contain more than 1,000 mgs of sodium. Foods to check carefully for the amount of salt/sodium include

- breakfast cereals

- lunch meats

- cheese

- bread

- crackers

FOOD LABEL GUIDE

% Daily Value shows how a food fits into a 2,000 calorie reference diet.

Daily Values are set by the government and based on current nutrition recommendations. Some labels list the daily values for a daily diet of 2,000 and 2,500 calories. Your own nutrient needs may be less or more.

Similar food products now have similar serving sizes to make comparisons easier. Serving sizes are based on amounts of food people actually eat.

Nutrient list covers those that are most important to your health.

Only two vitamins, A and C, and two minerals, calcium and iron, are required on food labels. Some food companies voluntarily list other vitamins and minerals found in their food.

Nutrition Facts
Serving Size 1 cup (228g)
Servings Per Container 2

Amount Per Serving

Calories 90   Calories from Fat 30

	% Daily Value*
	5%
	0%
Total Fat 3g	0%
Saturated Fat 0g	13%
Cholesterol 0mg	4%
Sodium 300mg	12%
Total Carbohydrate 13g	
Dietary Fiber 3g	
Sugars 3g	
Protein 3g	

Vitamin A 80%	•	Vitamin C 60%
Calcium 4%	•	Iron 4%

* Percent Daily Values are based on a 2,000 calorie diet. Your daily values may be higher or lower depending on your calorie needs:

	Calories:	2,000	2,500
Total Fat	Less than	65g	80g
Sat Fat	Less than	20g	25g
Cholesterol	Less than	300mg	300mg
Sodium	Less than	2,400mg	2,400mg
Total Carbohydrate		300g	375g
Dietary Fiber		25g	30g

Calories per gram:
Fat 9 • Carbohydrate 4 • Protein 4

Some labels tell the approximate number of calories in a gram of fat, carbohydrate and protein.

Note: Numbers on nutrition labels may be rounded.

- cookies

- sweets

Your doctor may be able to give you a list of foods to stay away from and foods to try to include in your diet.

Foods labeled "low sodium" may be a big help to you as you try to restrict your daily salt intake. So many people are on low-sodium diets today that food manufacturers now make foods with less salt. But even here, be careful to read the label yourself. What the food manufacturer defines as low sodium may contain far more sodium than you would like or that is good for you.

Heads-up at restaurants, too. Restaurant food tends to have more salt in it than your diet allows if you are salt-sensitive. When you eat out, ask for low-sodium or "heart-healthy" dishes. Your waiter will know what you mean because so many people ask for their food served this way. Ask, too, for salad dressings on the side so you can control how much you use, and ask for your main courses to be cooked without butter, in just a little olive oil. You'll be surprised at how easy it is to get better tasting, less fatty food from most restaurants you visit.

EAT FEWER SWEETS

Candy, cookies, soda, cakes and desserts should be eaten every once in awhile, not regularly. They are usually filled with calories, fat, sugar and salt but have almost no vitamins or minerals. That's why sweets are called "empty calorie" foods. They fill you up without giving you many of the vitamins and minerals you need. Over time, a diet that relies on cookies and sweets everyday strips a person of necessary vitamins and minerals, and can lead to a lack of these essential elements.

Soda pop is especially bad for us. It is packed with sugar, calories, and phosphate salts. The phosphate salts get in the way of our ability to absorb calcium, the mineral that makes our teeth and bones strong. Phosphate salts are especially hard on women, who generally do not get enough calcium, which helps prevent osteoporosis. Drink a soda pop of almost any kind and you will be filled up, but not with the better kind of food your body needs. All sweets are very hard on teeth too, especially children's teeth.

As you cut out sweets from your diet, you cut out calories and you will likely lose weight. That's good for your hypertension and for your health in general.

CUTTING DOWN ON SWEETS

If you want to cut back on eating sweets, start by getting them out of your house. Avoid any sweet that takes control over you. The kind you just can't stop eating. Try cutting back on sweets a little at a time. For a few weeks, cut out the cookies you eat every afternoon but continue to enjoy the piece of pie after dinner. Then, have the piece of pie three nights a week instead of every night. After a couple weeks, limit the pie to one special night a week. You will find you like it even more.

Eat fruit, fruit juice, low-sodium vegetable juice, dried fruits and whole-grain crackers instead of sweets.

You may find it surprisingly easy to cut back on sweets if you are exercising. Exercising has a way of "tuning up" the body. Your tastes may change as you exercise so that you begin to seek out the foods your body needs, like fruits and whole grain crackers.

If you have a very hard time cutting down on the amount of sweets you eat, tell your doctor, who may want to put you on vitamin and mineral supplements.

EATING FRUITS AND VEGETABLES

By cutting out canned and frozen vegetables and eating fresh ones instead, you not only will lower your sodium intake, you will increase the amount of vitamins, minerals, and fiber in your diet too.

Many vitamins and minerals are found in fresh vegetables and fruits with the brightest colors: dark green lettuce, collards and greens, broccoli, carrots, and oranges and yellow bananas, for example. If you are not already eating fresh foods, start slowly and work up to a diet that includes large servings of these foods each day.

Try them as snacks as you cut out cookies, potato chips, and candy.

VITAMIN SUPPLEMENTS

Because stress and certain blood pressure drugs can and do les-son, or deplete, the vitamins and minerals in the body, you may need to focus not only on diet but also on getting enough of the right vitamins. You can get these vitamins naturally from whole wheat and other whole grain products, but your doctor may also prescribe supplements. Commonly recommended supple-ments for those with hypertension are calcium, magnesium,

FIBER CONTENT OF FOODS

Foods	Portion	Fiber (grams)
peas, green	1/2 cup	5.2
kidney beans	1/2 cup	4.5
apple, with skin	1 small	3.9
apricots, with skin	2 medium	1.5
bread, whole wheat	1 slice	2.7
broccoli	1/2 cup	2.4
brown rice, cooked	1 cup	2.4
white rice, cooked	1 cup	2.4
lima beans	1/2 cup	1.4
lettuce	1/2 cup	0.5

and potassium, important minerals that aid in controlling blood pressure.

Your doctor may recommend vitamin supplements. Before you start a vitamin supplement plan, talk it over with your doctor. He or she can tell you about the possibilities and dangers of overdosing, and make sure that your vitamin schedule is in tune with your medical condition. Pregnant women must be especially careful about high vitamin intake.

NO FRYING

Heavily fried foods, which may taste so delicious, are so very unhealthy for us. They add a huge amount of unnecessary calories, and sometimes toxins, or poisons, as well. Oils for deep frying tend to change their chemistry when they are used more than once. The change is so great that our bodies recognize the oil and react against it as a toxic, or poisonous,

It is a good idea to avoid deep-fried foods.

substance. Remember that you're especially likely to run into these chemically changed fats in fast food restaurants.

For this and other reasons, it is a good idea to avoid deep-fried foods. Such foods should be eaten as a very special treat, maybe once or twice a year. Another reason to avoid very greasy foods is that, somehow, where there is grease there is salt!

At home, sautéing, steaming, baking, and microwaving with a small amount of safflower, canola, or olive oil can be done instead of frying.

Butter and lard should be used just a little, especially if you have heart disease or blood vessel damage along with your high blood pressure. Animal fats tend to speed clogging of the arteries. We want to go in the other direction, to begin eating and living in ways that will give our hearts and blood vessels the best chance to work properly.

To control hypertension by changing the way you eat means a lifelong promise to yourself. It does not require you to eliminate fat totally—simply, that you eat a balanced and healthy diet. You can eat the food you enjoy, and find wonderful flavor and zest in what you eat. Just be smart, and keep telling yourself that you are doing it for you and your family.

ALCOHOL

Your doctor may ask you to limit the amount of alcohol you drink. If you are in a social group that drinks, you may feel strange at first when you do not have a beer or drink with your friends. If they are good friends, tell them of your high blood pressure and ask for their support. If you cannot or do not

Tell your friends of your high blood pressure diagnosis and ask for their support.

want to tell them, you may want to think about the kind of friendship you have.

There are many other drinks you can choose including non-alcoholic beer, fruit juice, and low-sodium mineral water.

If any of this is terribly hard for you, if you find it difficult or impossible to stop drinking or to slow it down, you absolutely must get some help. It should not be hard for you or a big deal. If it is, you have a problem, called a substance abuse problem, and need help to work it out.

Keep in mind, too, that if you do drink at a bar, you'll probably want to have some of that bar food along with your drink. Forget it. It's usually filled with salt and calories.

SMOKING

If you smoke and have wanted to quit, now is the time. If you have high blood pressure, you should not smoke or live with anyone who smokes. *You and/or your spouse must quit.* Your doctor can tell you about the various products available to help you quit, such as nicotine chewing gum, patches, and hypnosis.

Nicotine is habit forming. It is highly addictive. Many who have quit or are trying to quit have formed support groups. Your doctor or your local lung association can tell you where to find support groups in your area. For more information, contact the American Cancer Society (http://www.cancer.org) or the American Lung Association (http:www.lungusa.org).

Though quitting is difficult, try not to get down on yourself. Remember that even if you have smoked all your life, quitting will make you healthier. After you stop, your lungs will start healing right away. Your chance of dying of a heart attack will be 50 percent less after you quit for one year. After five years, it is even less. After fifteen years, your chance of dying of lung cancer is the same as that of someone who never smoked. Your lungs will heal, you just have to give them a chance.

Your lungs will heal, you just have to give them a chance.

CONTROL YOUR WITHDRAWAL SYMPTOMS

Withdrawal Symptom	Things You Might Do Instead
Craving for cigarettes	Do something else; take slow, deep breaths; tell yourself, "Don't do it."
Anxiety	Take slow, deep breaths; don't drink caffeine drinks; do other things.
Irritability	Walk; take slow, deep breaths; do other things.
Trouble sleeping	Don't drink caffeine drinks in the evening; don't take naps during the day; imagine something relaxing like a favorite spot.
Lack of concentration	Do something else; take a walk.
Tiredness	Exercise; get plenty of rest.
Dizziness	Sit or lie down when needed; know that it will pass.
Headaches	Relax; take mild pain medication as needed.
Coughing	Sip water.
Constipation	Drink lots of water; eat high-fiber foods such as vegetables and fruits.
Hunger	Eat well-balanced meals; eat low-calorie snacks; drink cold water.

Reprinted from National Institute of Health, National Heart, Lung, and Blood Institute, "Nurses: Help Your Patients Stop Smoking," January 1993.

IN A NUTSHELL

- Taking medications on a regular schedule, changing your diet, and changing your lifestyle where necessary, may seem like major changes, but others have made these changes and been made happier by them. You can too.

- The power to change is in your hands, but you must be ready, knowing that the change will bring great benefits—including longer life.

- Starting on a regular exercise program may be the most important life-style change you make.

- For every person able to move a muscle, there is an appropriate exercise.

- A healthy diet can be just as tasty as one that damages your health.

- Diets heavy in salt, heavy in sweets, heavy in fast food and heavy in fried foods are dangerous diets.

- Fresh fruits and vegetables are good for you.

- Whole grains are good for you.

CHAPTER SEVEN

Stress Relief for Black Men and Women

As he dressed, Ronald Lloyd Lewis was still riding the wave of happiness that broke over him after his heart doctor, his cardiologist, said he could go home. Ronald had been in the hospital for five days recovering from a somewhat severe heart attack, and all that time he feared he'd have to undergo surgery. Now that Dr. Gant had studied Ronald's lab tests, he decided Ronald didn't need bypass surgery. "For what ails you, Ronald, medication will do the job. Untreated high blood pressure was part of the reason why you had the attack. Now, medication, along with a better diet and some work at reducing stress is what will keep you out of the surgeon's hands."

Ronald had never loved life so much as he did at this moment. It was a beautiful day, he was alive, his wife would be with him any moment, and he was going home. But he knew that if he wanted to keep all those good things, he would have to change his life.

Ronald was a very good lawyer who had also enjoyed political success. Just before he'd gotten ill, he worried a lot about whether to enter the race for congress, with the large demands it would make on his time and his money. And, of course, with one daughter in college and another close to entering, money was always on his mind. But greater even than those worries he knew deep down that the wild confidence he'd always enjoyed was a cover-up for something else: a feeling that he wasn't up to the job.

Ronald remembered how, after two hours of sleep, he had driven back from a late-night meeting and had been seized by a rush of adrenaline. Racing at speeds up to ninety-five miles per hour, he had passed everyone on the road, and when he finally pulled into the garage at three a.m. he had that feeling of victory. He'd won another race and he actually dreamed of the victory flag waving.

But now Ronald sensed that even while he was driving the car something else was driving him. He couldn't say at this stage of his life whether the roots of the problem were in his skin color or in something else altogether, and not knowing was one more layer of that same uneasiness he was feeling.

He knew enough about the history of how Black men are received in American politics to believe that skin color had a lot to do with his sense of inadequacy. But he also knew enough about human beings to see that, under all the masks that people wear to hide it, everyone had this fear of inadequacy. So the real question wasn't how to get rid of this feeling and this fear but how to tame the stress and use it to his advantage.

When he left Dr. Gant's office Ronald had already promised himself that he would learn the tricks of controlling that endlessly negative voice, and to get some peace from this inner stress at last.

What we can learn from Ronald's story

- *Stress and anger can make high blood pressure worse.*

- *Being Black in America can cause stress because of racial bias and intolerance in everyday life.*

- *You can cope with racial bias and learn ways to deal with it.*

- *Stress management plans, made together with your doctor, can help reduce high blood pressure.*

EVERYDAY STRESS

Thanks to research, we know a lot about stress today. For one thing, stress is a social evil that carries with it a heavy cost in terms of illness and loss of productivity. On a more human scale, stress means real physical suffering for many of us. For many more, it means that life has lost its zest because our experience comes to us through the screen of worry, or anxiety.

Everyday living, with oneself and with the problems associated with family, friends, and work, is stressful; no way around it. It comes with the territory for all of us—Black or white, rich or poor. So the question is, as Ronald Lewis wondered, how do we best learn to live with it?

Even people who seem relaxed and happy have stress in their lives. Often they are living with big problems. Because they have learned how to deal with stress, they're unlike that other group of people who live in constant anxiety, are quick to

> *Relaxed people manage the stress in their lives so that it rolls off of them like soft rain.*

anger, or frantic for that evening margarita.

Relaxed people manage the stress in their lives so that it rolls off of them like soft rain. Some of us seem to have been born knowing how to do this. Other people, and you can be one too, have taught themselves how to manage stress. You too can be one of those who don't sweat the small stuff and know how to handle the big stuff, too.

In this chapter we offer suggestions for reducing the harmful effects of stress on your life.

IDENTIFY THE STRESS

Your first job in dealing with stress is to identify when and why you are stressed. It's easy to point to the obviously irritating or annoying situations. You're in a hurry to get somewhere and the car in front of you stays at the stoplight after it has turned green. The driver is so wrapped up in his cell phone conversation that he's forgotten he's in a car. You honk, but he doesn't step on the gas. Or the shopkeeper keeps you standing while he's chatting endlessly with another customer. Or your husband comes home with a chip on his shoulder. You can complete the list.

But there may be other situations, less clear-cut, that make you feel stressed. Often, they build one on top of another. If it gets bad enough, you may come home at the end of every day feeling "stressed out."

Well, knowledge is power, especially when it's about yourself. Learn what sets you off. If you have trouble targeting the causes of your stress (professionals call these "stressors"), ask your spouse, close family, or best friends for their thoughts. You may be surprised at how readily they answer! They may say, "You are always stressed when you come back from one of those meetings," or "Since you've started that new commute you always look terrible when you get out of the car."

Identify the things that irritate you and begin to take control.

You may want to keep a stress diary for a week, jotting down the things that put your teeth on edge, and how you react to them. It's a way of getting to the root cause of the stress.

Going over your diary on the weekend, you may even find yourself laughing and saying, "Why did I ever react so strongly to such a small thing?" But even if you aren't laughing, once you know what irritates you, you can begin to take control.

HOW TO TURN STRESS AROUND

Many of us have learned to cope with the minor, day-to-day stressors. We accept them as irritations that we just deal with in the business of moving through life each day. We take a deep breath and move on. But there are always one or two silly situations that somehow get to us. They seem to have our name on them. Each time they happen, we go off like a grenade and, once again, we let them ruin our hour or even our day.

The next time you find yourself about to explode with anger

or rage, try to catch yourself. Take a moment to think before you act. Take control: make your thoughts positive or try a bit of humor.

Laughter is one of the best cures for stress. Go ahead, make fun of the situation. This way, you save your energy for the big events in your life that really deserve your attention. That's one of the problems with constant stress: we can spend so much time on small irritations that we have little or nothing left to put toward our bigger, serious problems and, for that matter, our serious pleasures. We "burn out" on the little things. Laughter helps us see the truth: That small problems are just that—small.

When Ron started keeping a stress diary, he saw that bad drivers sent his mind reeling down its own bad road. A bad driver he met on the road instantly stood for everything that was wrong with Ron's world. "Of course this is happening to me," Ron would think. "Things will never go my way, they never do." It was as if someone had placed bad drivers in his path in order to annoy him. It was as if everyone was against Ron. Once that feeling took over, Ron was sunk. He felt terrible about himself and about the world. All because of one bad driver!

After his heart attack, Ron started to experiment. When he met a bad driver he reminded himself it had nothing to do with him. He thought about all the other people the driver would meet that day. He laughed about all the irritation and chaos that one bad driver would cause. And with that laughter, Ron was on the road to living his life better.

This "irritation mode" happens to many of us. The more we slip into this frame of mind, the more harm we do to ourselves, in mind, body, and spirit. And the opposite is true: the more we take control and remember not to take little issues so seriously and personally, the stronger we grow in mind, body and spirit.

Here are a few other tips for dealing with "on the spot" stress:

Practice deep and steady breathing when you are faced with stress. This calms the body and the mind. Count your breaths as a way to slow and steady your breathing. There isn't enough research for us to say that relaxation techniques definitely lower blood pressure. We do know that they can reduce the hold that stress has on us.

If you feel yourself tensing up, slowly relax the muscles that are tense. Start with your jaw and move to your shoulders, back, arms, and legs. You'll be surprised how your mood can change.

Smiling works too. It's an odd trick the body has. Think of something funny or happy and allow yourself to smile over it. If we try to be happy or to think happy thoughts happiness tends to follow. Try it.

If you've had a very stressful experience, take a quick break and go for a walk outside or through the hallways of your office. Immediately changing your location can do wonders for helping you to let go of what happened. Let your body help you shake off the stress. When you walk, you will take in more oxygen and when you move your arms and legs, you will start to calm your body and mind. Allow your mind to come to grips with the stressful situation. But limit the time. After a few minutes, make your mind focus on what you see around you, the people, the trees, the business of the day. You will start to relax. You may find walks like this amazingly refreshing. If you really want to get away from your problems, go to a park where there are children. Watching them play and hearing them laugh can be terrific medicine. Or if you can't find children, watch some guys playing basketball in the corner park. Or look at a puppy playing. That too can ease your mind and lower your stress level.

RELAXING AS PART OF YOUR LIFE

Sometimes our lives can get so busy, so demanding, and so downright stressful that we no longer do those activities that we used to do for fun and that helped us relax. Without knowing it, we may sometimes cut ourselves off from the very activities that keep our lives less stressful and our blood pressure low.

Know what activities give you enjoyment and relaxation.

Know what activities are enjoyable and relaxing. Make a list of the top ten. Maybe they are things you used to do but have stopped doing. Never mind. Write them down. Everyone's list will be different. Yours might include

- sitting quietly and listening to music

- playing sports

- gardening

- dancing

- singing in the choir

- bible study or teaching Sunday School class

- playing a musical instrument or singing, alone or with friends

- reading mystery novels

- cooking

- shooting pool

- just walking around the neighborhood and taking in the sights

Make your list and then start doing the activity again. No time for it? Make the time. Make it because it is good for you. You have our permission! Now give yourself your own. Remember that the time you put into learning, or re-learning, to relax is time your friends and family will thank you for, because they'll see the change. And you may well enjoy the added benefit of seeing your blood pressure go down.

EXERCISE

For many people, exercise is a great way to let go of stress. A walk during lunch hour or after work, a swim at the pool, or a game of basketball has a way of refreshing the mind and relaxing the body. As we've seen, exercise is a very effective way to lower blood pressure.

As an change from traditional exercise, there is yoga. There are many books and tapes on this subject. Yoga may help you learn to focus, free your mind of worries, and relax and stretch your muscles.

Massage therapy could be of benefit. There are licensed massage therapists in most states. There are even classes at local community centers across the country that teach you how to give massages.

CREATE!

Creative pastimes and hobbies feed the soul in a unique way and help us get back to our true selves. They also give us some control that may be lacking in other areas of our life. (This is also true of exercise.) Often, when we tend to our creative life, the rest of our life seems to go better. Find a creative activity that suits you. Take a drawing class. Learn to knit or do carpentry. Learn to cook. Play the guitar or another musical instrument. Get together with a group of friends and form a writing group. Be creative, get involved!

SOCIALIZE

The worst way to suffer stress is alone. Stress can mean total self involvement, depression, and feelings that you're not worth anything. That's why people suffering stress often pull away from family and friends. Or their hostile behaviors may drive others away. But we *are* social animals, after all, and there are a number of ways to restart our friendships and contact with others. Here are a few:

Call friends to have a meal together. We all know how easy it is to be unhappy when the phone doesn't ring. Well, sometimes you can snap out of your sense of isolation simply by contacting others. An evening with friends can remind you of how much the give and take with others can improve your mood.

Keep a pet. This has its own special rewards. The love you give to your pet takes you away from your own problems and makes you focus on another being. Studies have shown that pets such as cats, dogs and birds can reduce the stress in your life, bring you happiness, and help you live longer.

Sometimes, too, when stress overwhelms you, talking with others can help you see the issue more clearly and put it into perspective. Remember that many times, when we go through stress, it's not advice that we need. Simply by talking it out, we may begin to see a way out of it.

TALK IT OUT

In the same way get into the habit of saying what you think, knowing what you want, and doing what's in your power to get it. This doesn't mean you have to become a loudmouth or a bully. It means you must have self-respect. As you express your views, you'll find that others will express theirs to you. You may find yourself changing, or others changing as you guide them. Start

Get into the habit of saying what you think, knowing what you want, and doing what's in your power to get it.

conversations. Begin friendships. You may be out of practice and feel rusty. But, as in all walks of life, practice will make things, if not perfect, better. It's just a question of trying.

STRESS AT WORK

Stress on the job, as we've seen, is a big problem. And sometimes you can't do much about it. A dead-end job, doing the same thing day after day, under a bullying (or, sometimes, sexist or racist) boss can be a true nightmare. Sometimes there's nothing else to do but to learn new skills or sharpen the ones you have and look for a new job.

But often you can make things better for yourself. For most people, what causes stress on the job is the feeling that they have no power. Where possible, then, be an active citizen in the workplace. Ask questions and make suggestions. And start to build good relationships with co-workers. Sometimes that sense of togetherness can be the beginning of a new sense of control.

Experts urge you to be make decisions and be forceful at work. How do I get there from here? you may ask. Simply writing down what the problem is and a list of the options you have for solving it—even the option of doing nothing—can be an excellent start. List not only the solutions that stand out but also the hidden ones; and for each, list its pros and cons.

> *Action is nearly always preferable to inaction.*

Sometimes, through such steps, you find the problems that seemed to have no answers actually have several. Play with them, keeping in mind that if you choose one and it doesn't pay off, you can turn to another.

Merely working toward a solution will bring its own rewards. Action, in such matters, is almost always better than inaction, or doing nothing, and clear and patient thought can be a form of action.

Knowing clearly what you want is the first step toward getting it. Sometimes we sink so deeply into stress-related depression that we feel too powerless to want anything. In that state any action is difficult. To get things going again, try making a list of ten things you like to do. Make other lists of things you'd like to see happen in your life. Stay focused and keep your eyes on the big picture—even when, as Dr. Martin Luther King, Jr. put it, "the cup of endurance runs over."

SLEEP

If you're sleepless because of stress, you need to correct the problem. Sleeplessness feeds stress and makes you moody, angry, more likely to become ill. Regulating your sleep should be a top priority.

That means staying away from stimulants, things like alcohol, caffeine, and nicotine, which will keep you awake and disrupt sleep. Learn good habits for getting ready to sleep. If you watch a violent movie before going to bed, you're not likely to slip easily into sleep. Find ways to calm yourself before bed. Read something that soothes or makes you feel good. Read your Bible or Sunday school lesson. Listen to mellow music.

Once in bed, remove the clear obstacles to sleep. Use earplugs to keep out annoying noise. Relax your body by regularly tensing and then relaxing your muscles—first your feet, then gradually work up your legs, the trunk of your body, your chest, neck, jaw, cheeks and brow. Tense and relax your muscles a few times if you need to. It works.

Pay attention to your breathing. Try to steady and slow it. When your mind wanders, bring it back, gently, to the in and out of your breath.

If none of this helps, other help is available. Ask your doctor to refer you to a sleep clinic where you can get medical treatment or treatment through biofeedback. If you are suffering sleep problems, self-medication with over-the-counter drugs can be risky. Best talk to your doctor.

MEDITATION

Meditation is an important spiritual practice for managing stress. Millions of Americans have found it a useful exercise that calms the spirit and allows them to taste life's fruits more fully. These days, in major cities, meditation centers are easy to find, and many of them offer free or low cost lessons. The basic principles, or guidelines, of meditation are simple enough, however, and you can begin them on your own.

Pick a time of day and a place that's fairly quiet and free from people or events that might distract or interrupt you. Sit on a thick cushion on the floor, legs crossed, or in a straight-backed chair. Keep an upright posture so that your back is not up against the back of the chair. Your spine, your neck, and the top of your head should all be in a line, as though someone were pulling you up with a string attached to the top of your head. In other words, sit tall.

Sit still, resting your hands palms down on your thighs. Rest your eyes also. Look at a point about five feet ahead of you on the floor. Keep your eyes there but gently, without fixing your focus. Find and feel your breathing in your abdomen. You can do this by pushing your breath all the way out when you breathe out and then sending your awareness to the in-and-out of your breath. Do this for ten or so breaths, until you've found your breathing. Then just breathe naturally, without trying to breathe in any special way, but being aware of your breathing as it goes in and out on its own.

You might begin meditating by sitting for ten minutes a day, or ten minutes twice a day, and then lengthen the time as you get used to the practice. Set a timer so you don't need to watch the clock. It is more important to continue to practice from day to day than to sit for longer periods of time. For example, sit for ten minutes every day when you get up rather than sitting for thirty minutes on Monday and then not getting back to it until Thursday.

You will notice as you sit that your mind throws off an endless stream of images, worries, plans, daydreams, and thoughts, both good and bad. They race in, one after another. In the beginning you may be shocked by the power of your mind's energy. This is what the Buddhist's call "monkey mind" or "grasshopper mind"—for reasons that are clear.

But meditation trains the mind to think of this endless stream as a passing show, no one thought more important than another. When you find yourself getting caught up in your plans for the day, whether an appointment, worry about your children, meal plans, vacation plans, or fantasies, just label this as "thinking," and return your focus to your breathing and to the present moment. This will happen over and over in the course of ten minutes. Just keep starting over, going back to the breathing and bringing yourself back to the present.

The point is to stay alert and relaxed, letting thoughts come and go. Meditation is sometimes falsely looked at as a way to "clear your mind" You will not clear it, but you will learn to look at it in a different way—accepting all the parts of your mind, the "good" thoughts and the "bad" ones, with balance and calm.

SUPPORT GROUPS

Much of what we've been talking about has to do with fighting stress through our own efforts. But sometimes our problems become more than we can handle alone. That's when, blessedly, we can turn to professionals to help us. For example, we highly recommend twelve-step programs such as Alcoholics Anonymous and similar programs that can help us kick bad habits and heal us of the shame that helped make us dependent in the first place.

In a support group you can share your most painful feelings of shame, guilt, and stress without losing face. When you listen to the moving and sometimes heroic stories of others it helps put your situation into perspective. You will find many people "worse" off than you, so there is no reason to be embarrassed! Support groups can be very helpful.

These days almost everyone can find a support group. Many of us have found that being able to laugh freely, and cry with others, is in itself good medicine. It can be the beginning of a return to the social world.

PROFESSIONAL THERAPY

When all else fails, there is professional therapy and help. Your doctor or your minister can recommend a counselor who can help. Sometimes a few sessions do the job, by shifting your focus that half-inch you need to bring you back to a better life. Sometimes it takes longer.

Therapy is there for you. It's a tool for your benefit. Don't wait to use it. Not enough Black people have learned to reap the benefits of such therapy. Let's change that, starting now, starting with you. If you've seriously tried other means of stress relief and found that they didn't work, try therapy. It has worked for many and can work for you.

Our basic theme is simple, and we'll repeat it one more time to be sure that it's clear: *No one has to be driven over the edge of despair by stress, anger, fear, racism, or self-doubt. Help is available!*

Although we have suggested strategies for relieving stress that have worked for many people, we don't wish to make the problem seem too simple. Life is often unfair and being Black in America is usually stressful. "Living under the veil," as Dr. W. E. B. Dubois said, is all too real for many of us. At times, the stress of everyday life can seem more than we can bear. That is why we must hold in mind not only the strategies, or actions, we've listed in this chapter but also that old but powerful saying, "The day we did things right was the day we stood up to fight. Keep your eyes on the prize and hold on." Your good health is a prize worth fighting for.

IN A NUTSHELL

- The first step toward managing stress is to know what is bothering you is

- You can manage stress by:
  - thinking positively and having a sense of humor
  - practicing deep, calm breathing
  - relaxing your muscles
  - walking or doing other forms of regular exercise
  - getting together with friends
  - participating in healthy forms of recreation
  - getting a good night's sleep
  - practicing your spirituality alone or in support groups

- When you need it, professional help is available.

CHAPTER EIGHT

Prayer and Healing

From Dr. Galen's view, Curtis Starrett was an ideal patient. Curtis came to Dr. Galen after a yearly checkup at work showed Starrett's blood pressure was way too high. He was eager to start treatment. His father had suffered a stroke at forty-two and Curtis's mother was left to raise five boys. So Curtis knew the costs of uncontrolled hypertension.

At forty-eight, Curtis had recently remarried and had two young children at home. They were his pride and joy. "I have to be there for them," he told the doctor, and it was clear he meant it. Curtis was glad to start on medication, stopped visiting the lunch truck at work, and instead ate the low-salt, low-fat lunches his wife made for him. After four months, Curtis's pressure came down but not as much as he and the doctor had hoped. It was during that visit, as he and Dr. Galen were talking about what to do next, that Curtis said, "Doc, if I die suddenly from my pressure, I don't think I'll go to heaven."

Oddly, that deep thought surprised Curtis. He hadn't gone to church for some years—in fact, not since his bitter divorce from his first wife. Before that, he had been a deeply spiritual man who prayed often. But now, as he felt his life to be on the scales, in balance with his death, phrases he used to hear and feel in church rang in his head: "Ever have any doubt? The Lord will surely bring you out!. . . . He will never let you down. . . ." And he'd always gotten great comfort from this passage in Proverbs: Trust in the Lord with all thine heart; and lean not unto thine own understanding. In all thy ways acknowledge Him and He shall direct thy paths."

Thinking about all this now, Curtis shared with Dr. Galen that he believed he was spiritually "not lined up" with God. When Dr. Galen pressed him on this, Curtis told him, "I feel that I'm in a kind of double bind. During that terrible time of the divorce, with all my anger and loss, I thought I wasn't worthy of God's love. But there was another side of it, too. I felt that God had left me."

Dr. Galen felt that Curtis wanted to talk with God but was afraid. He encouraged Curtis to get back to a congregation. He told him bluntly what he saw, that Curtis was a spiritual man who had been ignoring this part of himself. Now, for his health—physical and spiritual—he needed to make up with God. "You know, Curtis, I'm convinced that if you can do that, you'll feel more peace at home and at work—in short, that you'll feel less stressed."

Two months later, when Curtis came back for a check-up, he had a lot to say. He *had* gone back to church, he said, and as he felt accepted and forgiven by God it had lifted a great load off his shoulders. Even before he took Curtis's blood pressure, Dr. Galen noted that Curtis was calmer than he'd ever seen him. When he took Curtis's blood pressure the numbers agreed. Curtis's blood pressure was almost normal.

What we can learn from Curtis's story

- *The mind-body connection is real.*

- *Practicing your religion can help lower your blood pressure.*

- *Start attending church or participating in other social groups where you can share your feelings and improve the spiritual side of your life.*

- *Prayer can help you feel better in both body and spirit.*

STRESS AND PRAYER

Black men and women have a long history of turning to God to help ease stress and doubts, to answer the hard questions, and to get sympathy and wisdom. So for many of us praying regularly, and feeling connected to a higher power, is the right kind of medicine to help keep blood pressure low.

> *A relaxed and peaceful state of mind has a positive, calming effect on the body.*

As you learned from the chapter on stress, the body truly tenses up during stress and releases certain hormones that help us rise to the challenge before us. The opposite also happens. A relaxed and peaceful state of mind has a positive, calming effect on the body as well.

The cardiologist Dr. Randolph C. Byrd reports that patients

who pray daily are less likely to be sick than those who do not pray, and, if they become sick, the sickness will be less severe ("Positive Therapeutic Effects of Intercessory Prayer in a Coronary Care Unit Population." *Southern Medical Journal* 81:7 [1998].) Other researchers have found that prayer can reduce high blood pressure and headaches, ease anxiety and stress, and even help heal wounds. Dozens of studies show the positive effect of prayer.

At the simplest level, prayer helps us to slow down and relax, something many of us must learn to do in this stressful world. But prayer also works at a deeper level. To keep in contact with a higher power is to know that we do not carry the weight of the world alone but can share that load. Such contact prepares us to be fully worthy of our existence here, by letting us be open to the joys and challenges of the world, and in that way make of our lives a kind of thanksgiving.

The relaxed feeling we have when we pray, meditate, or sing in church happens because we are willing to put our troubles in God's hands. In prayer or meditation we say, "Lord I don't know what will happen but I know that in Your hands I will be all right."

Following a spiritual path leads us to understanding, faith, and God's love. And that becomes the source of calm, peace, and confidence that change for the better is within our reach. In such a state, we tend to have lower blood pressure.

HOW BEST TO PRAY

For those who are ready to believe, prayer will work its healing. Pray each day if you can. Choose a time when you can be alone, perhaps after you wake in the morning. Choose a quiet place that holds meaning for you, perhaps kneeling by the side of your bed, or sitting in a chair in your room. A church or mosque near your work is most likely open at the noon hour for the many people who want to pray. Find it. Go in.

Pray for strength, for peace, for healing. Pray not only for yourself but for those you love.

Pray each day if you can. Choose a time when you can be alone.

If anger and stress—distress— seem to be driving your life, tell God about this. It can be a first step toward seeing the destructive forces that threaten you. As the songs say, why not bring your burdens to God and lay them down? That's when you can know what so many others have known: the balm and comfort that come to us when we find a living spiritual connection.

Once you have felt that comfort, it will be easy for you to ask God for help in controlling your blood pressure, for guidance in relearning how to relax and enjoy life, for the strength to exercise and to stick to a low-salt diet, to quit smoking or any other of the many ways that we know will help us live healthier lives.

Pray and ask God to bless your medicine and treatments and give thanks for them.

Remember, many doctors today know the healing power of prayer. Plan with your doctor how to include faith in God and prayer as part of your treatment, a part so important that you also make it part of your doctor visit.

RECOVERING YOUR SPIRITUALITY

Bring back those religious or spiritual traditions that were important to you. Sometimes, simple things work best. If meal-time prayer was very important to you, bring it back and see how good it feels. Some families find joy in reading aloud to each other their favorite passages from the Bible. Other families share with each other every night where they saw God's work during the day. Maybe your best memories were of singing hymns with your family. What's holding you back? Start singing. If there's no time after dinner, sing with the kids as you drive them to school.

STRENGTH FROM THE SCRIPTURES

Many passages in the Bible talk about stress and its relief. Jesus offered rest, relief of heavy burdens, and peace of mind to those who cast their cares upon God. The apostle Paul described this as peace "which passes all understanding and it shall keep your hearts and minds through Christ Jesus."

The Bible is full of paths to that peace. Many people call on the Psalms, and the twenty-third Psalm is a favorite of many faced with difficulty, small and great. Of course, you know it, but here it is for you to reflect on:

> The Lord is my shepherd, I shall not want. He makes me
> lie down in green pastures. He leads me beside still waters.
> He restores my soul. He leads me in paths of righteousness
> for His name's sake. Even though I walk through the valley
> of the shadow of death, I fear no evil, for Thou art with me,
> Thy rod and Thy staff they comfort me. Thou preparest a

table before me in the presence of my enemies. Thou anointest my head with oil, my cup overflows. Surely goodness and mercy shall follow me all the days of my life, and I shall dwell in the house of the Lord forever. Amen.

Here are other passages you may also want to refer to for comfort in distress:

Philippians 4: 6-7: "Have no anxiety about anything but in everything by prayer and supplication with thanksgiving let your requests be made known to God. And the peace of God, which passes all understanding, will keep your hearts and minds in Christ Jesus."

Isaiah 26:3: "Thou dost keep him in perfect peace, whose mind is stayed on thee, because he trusts in thee."

Proverbs 17:22 wisely says that being merry and happy is like a medicine for us. The scriptures also state that we should not allow the day to be completed with us remaining angry.

Mind, body, and spirit are connected. Hebrews 4:12, discusses those rich connections, and explains why it is impossible to divide one from another. We are speaking of a living power here:

"For the word of God is living and active, sharper than any two-edged sword, piercing to the division of soul and spirit, of joints and marrow, and discerning the thoughts and intentions of the heart."

CONGREGATIONS

The sharing that comes from being part of a congregation, Bible study group or meditation group can bring tremendous benefits, socially, spiritually, and physically.

Other Helpful Scriptures

Joshua 1:9	Help
Psalm 23	Help, certainty of death
Psalm 27:14	When facing difficulty
Psalm 34:19	When suffering illness
Psalm 46	To face a crisis
Psalm 49:15	Certainty of death
Psalm 91	Facing illness
Isaiah 40	When discouraged
Ephesians 6	Equipment for difficulties
Timothy 2	Major difficulties
Hebrews 11	Trust in God

Spiritual engagement is vitally important to health.

Prayer can bring us into a larger network of belief and practice, into community and into service. Such spiritual engagement is vitally important to health.

Study after study shows that being alone fits hand in glove with stress. Being part of a religious community can lead to greater gifts of self and ties to others. Attending a church and getting involved in Sunday school or in other forms of service are ways of connecting with something bigger and more important than yourself.

Again, scientific research backs this up. Studies show that during church services, the effect of many people worshipping and praising God together causes the release of substances in the brain and body that can greatly lessen the sense of pain and illness.

But the important thing isn't whether we look at this from a scientific or a spiritual angle. Knowing that we are loved by God and part of His community can help calm us and lower blood pressure. Being part of a congregation gives us strength to make the changes we need to make. Struggle is part of the human condition and church is the place we are reminded of this. God and our fellow worshippers give us strength to tackle our problems.

You may be a member of a congregation in which the "laying on of hands" and anointing with oil is practiced. This practice is a part of the Church service designed for persons who are sick or have physical ailments and need healing. Such practices can play an important role in healing and are perfectly in line with the treatments you may be getting from your doctor.

HEALING AND SPIRITUAL TEACHINGS

Some people feel that once they have been spiritually helped they are healed forever. We've seen patients with high blood pressure and other health problems stop their medications because they believed that taking medicine conflicts with God's teachings. Don't go that way. For the Spirit to act within you, you must hold up your

Use your own spiritual strength and the strength of your congregation to help your medicine work.

end. In that way, you let the power of the spirit help you heal. Use your own spiritual strength and the strength of your congregation to help your medicine work.

When we are ill or struggling with high blood pressure, we have a contract with our Maker to do our part to help heal our bodies and keep ourselves well. One way to think of medicine is that health care providers are human instruments that God uses to help us achieve the highest levels of health. Our bodies are temples, God's temples, and when we take care of them we are being respectful to God. In the words of I Corinthians 6: 19-20: "Do you not know that your body is the temple—the very sanctuary—of the Holy Spirit who lives within you, whom you have received from God?"

Inviting the power of God into health issues can bring dramatic improvements to you—and sometimes complete healing.

IN A NUTSHELL

- Regular spiritual practice is good for your body and your soul.

- If you've lost the habit of going to your place of worship, now is a good time for you to start going again.

- Religion and spiritual practice offer a place where you can put your burdens down.

SOME LAST WORDS

Most of us learn along the road of life to take good care of the things that mean the most to us. We put oil in the car, replace the brake linings when they're worn, and do whatever it takes to keep the car running and to give it a long life. In the same way, if we own a house, we take care of it. If it needs a roof, we put up new shingles, because we know that if we let the roof go much more damage will follow.

Our body is our car and our home. It too needs our attention and care. Eating a healthy diet and avoiding the substances that harm the body are important parts of the care. So are regular visits to the doctor and religiously taking the medications your doctor prescribes. So too is exercise, without which your body, much like a car that's kept in the garage for too long, simply doesn't run well—and may not run at all.

But of course, it's not that simple. Your body also responds to psychological pressures. In this book we've tried to help you better understand stress. You don't need our help to *feel* stress, but to understand the sources of stress, as you've learned, is to help cope with it.

Finally, your body is not just a physical and psychological instrument. It is also a spiritual vessel. We believe—and there is a lot of evidence to support the view—that an active spiritual life is good for your heart because spiritual involvement takes some of the burdens of life off your back. Certainly, we don't pray to God simply because prayer can help us control our blood pressure, but that can be one of the many ways prayer can help us: Sustaining the temple of the body that has been given us.

If you use what you learned in this book to change your lifestyle, the good results will show themselves as your blood pressure comes down and you are better able to cope with stressful events. Finally, the end results will show in the numbers. African Americans, Black people in general, have the same right to good health that all human beings do. We hope this book helps you find your way to those benefits.

APPENDIX ONE

Questions About Hypertension to Ask Your Doctor

How serious is my problem?

What do I have to do to control my blood pressure?

Do I need to buy a monitoring device?

What do I do if I take the medicine, exercise, and watch my diet, and still my blood pressure goes up?

Can you tell me a place where I could get training in stress management?

Is my medication covered by Medicare or Medicaid?

How much exercise should I do, and what kind of exercise would be best for me?

Can you give me any information about the kind of diet that would work for me and help lower my blood pressure?

INDEX